What Others Say About Shangrila Rendon & Feisty Fox Coaching

"Prepared Beyond Expectations"

Thank you Coach Shangrila! I'm grateful for your patience and coaching. You prepared me better than I realized.

– Dr. Mona-Lisa Pinkney, Sr. Director at Nike, Oregon

"Lessons from Resilience"

Shangrila has bared herself in order to find her own authenticity and has wisely chosen to gather the lessons learned along the road that is sadly too-often traveled so that others may benefit. I have witnessed first-hand Shangrila's resilience, determination, passion and athleticism and I believe in her mission.

– Steve King, Author, Voice of Ultraman, Counselor and Athlete, British Columbia

"Life-Changing Guidance"

Her guidance with the training... It taught me so many life lessons not only in running but all the principles I've learned, I have applied in other areas of my life and I just feel that it made me a better person, a stronger person, not just physically, but emotionally, mentally, and also spiritually. It just influenced my life in different dimensions that I really honestly didn't expect would be possible.

– Julie Uychiat, Director of Clinical Services, Abbott World Marathon Majors, World Marathon Challenge, Marathon de Sables Finisher, Arizona

"A Coach Who Inspires"

Coach Shangrila bares her soul in moving recount of how anything is possible w/ honest self-reflection, grit and determination. Through her coaching, she pours out immense energy, heart, and kindness to students of all levels, inspiring her students to be not only better athletes but better people.

– Katy Freitag, Lawyer, Owner of Bloomquist Law Firm, USAT Nationals Qualifier, IM Qualifier, Texas

"Loving Triathlon Again"

I can't say enough about Feisty Fox Coaching. It has truly made swimming, biking, and running fun again. I am blessed to be a part of an amazing group of coaches and athletes... I was skeptical. I thought it was going to be a one-size-fits-all program, but it was not... Needed guidance, needed to be accountable, needed to learn to train smarter, needed to bring back my passion for the sport... My goal, to beat my time from last year. Their training is based on you, your lifestyle, and your time schedule. It WAS NOT a one-size-fits-all... Not only am I loving triathlons again, but I am also happy, I smile through my races and my training, it's not painful, and I recover.

– Jax Grave, IM Kona Finisher, business owner, Hawaii

"Waking Up Pain-Free"

What an incredible experience! I went in laser-focused on getting coached on nutrition to help in my first official-in person 70.3, but with an open mind that things may differ from what I've been doing. GOT way more out of the program! For starters, I got small improvements on my nutrition, but got help with my mindset after a 10-week injury, improvements in my running form, my biking form, & swimming technique. Got lessons in taking care of my body & learning a few tricks/strategies as well.

One of the best things I got (which wasn't even part of my goals) was waking up pain-free every morning. Not 1 muscle/joint was hurting & I have NEVER felt like that!... Definitely a shortcut to all the errors in training & strategies...I wish I had done this sooner instead of having to learn the hard way on my own!

– Paul Edward Rodriguez, Engineer, Michigan

"They Truly Care About Every Athlete"

I recommend the coaching services of Feisty Fox Coaching because of their sheer dedication to their athletes. Everything from compiling the data of workouts and evaluating it to their abundance of support, they truly care about each and every athlete.

– Daniel Kohuth, Alaska

"Finally Got Over Water Anxiety"

Coach Shangrila was so helpful. I had a diving incident 12 years ago and honestly had true anxiety putting my face in the water. Coach really helped me get past that! Thank you.

– Amanda Bright, Physician Assistant, Kentucky

"Becoming The Best Version Of Myself"

Feisty Fox Coaching embodies this quote: 'Coaching is unlocking a person's potential to maximize their growth.' Coach Shangrila's belief in my abilities has been a powerful driving force in my journey to becoming the best version of myself... I am absolutely thrilled to continue this incredible journey as I prepare for the Ironman California.

– Gaye, Physical Therapist, California

"I Was a Bit Skeptical..."

I recently completed the 30-day swim bootcamp. At first, I was a bit skeptical because I've never done virtual coaching.

However, I soon realized that the training was top-notch. I had multiple coaches checking in each day to see how things were going. I had access to a plethora of useful information. I was in direct contact with the head coach almost every day. All my questions were answered within 24 hours or less! The improvements that I made in that 30 days were monumental and invaluable. The overall quality and value were definitely worth it.

– Mark Kramer, Michigan

"Back to Triathlon After 8 Years"

I hadn't competed in 8 years and decided to jump in with both feet! I joined the Triathlon Boot Camp and literally hit the ground running as my first competition was only 4 weeks away...

Through Feisty Fox Coaching, I have come to understand all of the aspects of becoming a better, faster, stronger, injury-free athlete... Thank you Feisty Fox Coaches for helping me PR in my first triathlon in 8 years and complete a seriously difficult OWS... I have only just begun!!

– Kat, Hawaii

"Mastered The Art Of Teaching"

I couldn't recommend Coach Shangrila G. Rendon and the Feisty Fox Team enough—the swim boot camp coaching program is excellent and easy to follow from beginners to advanced triathletes.

She is an accomplished coach who really knows her subject and has mastered the art of teaching... She has a great team of coaches and Shangrila is always around to answer questions, solve problems, and motivate when needed.

– Patricia Kolias, Massachussets, Ironman Kona Finisher

"From Barely Running to Marathon Finisher"

I would 100% recommend to anyone. Went from barely able to run a quarter of a mile on June 1 to marathon finisher on Oct 15!!

Was crazy challenging but had a great clear plan with lots of support (even with the online program!) Shangrila always had a positive happy attitude which made you want to keep going even when times were tough and would adjust the training plan to unexpected life events!

– Tina B, ER Doctor, Marathoner, California

"Phenomenal Support"

Excellent video analysis and customized training. Phenomenal support from the coaching team and other more experienced athletes.

You will have the opportunity to meet and listen to subject matter experts in running, swimming, nutrition, psychology, and more. It has been the best experience in my life in terms of sports coaching. Five-star rating!

– Tudor Gradea, Engineer, Texas

"I Had No Clue How Online Coaching Could Work"

I'm so happy I stumbled upon Coach Shangrila and Feisty Fox Coaching! A friend talked me into competing in a triathlon and I got into my own workout routine. But being the competitor that I am, I wanted to do better. Coach Shangrila has given me that ability.

I have worked with her for a year now... all of my times are better. And more important, I am a stronger athlete!

I had no clue how online coaching could work. It's awesome! I workout on my time schedule and Coach is always there with me (I hear her in my head giving critical feedback!) I'm constantly telling my friends about Feisty Fox training!

– Kelly Rock Lakia, Veterinararian, 70.3 & USAT National Finisher, Indiana

"I Tried Everything"

I finished my first triathlon (IM 70.3 Santa Cruz) last year but I knew I had to improve swimming. I tried other online programs as well as apps and some were good but none of them provided feedback. Swim instructors I worked with didn't have a triathlon background.

After I worked with Coach Shangrila G. Rendon, I improved my breathing pattern and got better at swimming.

– Alpesh Parmar, California

"Break Out Of a Plateau"

I had a great experience with Feisty Fox Coaching. If you are looking to break out of a plateau, improve your form and speed, this could be a game-changer for you!

It definitely takes a commitment, not just to getting the swim workouts done, but to be actively engaged in the process by studying the materials provided and providing timely, thorough feedback. If you are willing to make the commitment, you should definitely be able to see the results!

– Stephanie Gordon, Washington

"I Got My Old Self Back!"

Feisty Fox Coaching has helped me get my fitness back! After 8 years of being inactive due to childbirth complications, I was finally able to get my old self back, and I think I am in better shape now than I was before.

When I tried to self-train, I thought that I would never be able to get stronger or faster again because my body just couldn't handle the workouts. I was wrong! With Coach Shangrila's guidance, I am now faster and stronger. With her structured workouts, she makes sure that you progress at the right pace so you don't get injured. Thanks, Feisty Fox Coaching!

– Pillar, California

"I Thought I Was Already Doing Everything..."

I didn't know what I was missing until I joined Feisty Fox Coaching. I thought I was already doing everything I needed for myself and my body until I joined. It turns out I really needed a lot of help and guidance!

There isn't any other coach or group I would trust with helping me achieve my goals. The Feisty Fox team and community has been such a GREAT resource these past months.

I've truly learned more about myself and how to better myself as an athlete. Coach Shangrila, Coach Jeff, Coach Vineta, and everyone else have been amazing, and I love working with them!

– Vivian Justin Coloma, California

"Life-Changing Results"

I took the leap and did the 30-day Swim Bootcamp and I can honestly say it was life-changing. I went from just sort of trying out triathlon training to truly feeling like an athlete...

In 30 days I learned more than the last 10 years of trying to figure it out on my own. I also became more efficient, gained endurance, and increased my CSS speed... I was so impressed after 30 days that I signed on for more training.

– Andrea Wilson, Missouri

"Push Me Just Enough Without Overdoing It"

Feisty Fox coaching has been amazing and ESSENTIAL throughout my training! They really know how to push me just enough without overdoing it, and their advice on everything from technique to pacing has been a game-changer... Having someone keep me on track and motivated has made a huge difference. I honestly don't think I'd have made it this far without their help!

– Cedric Escay, California

"Finally Achieving My Triathlon Dream"

A long time ago, I had a dream to finish a sprint triathlon. I didn't know how to do so.

Coach Shangrila and the Feisty Fox community gave me the opportunity to start this amazing journey—not only to challenge myself to do better but also by increasing my well-being in an unimaginable manner. They offer the exact tools for you, not only for taking care of workouts but for taking care of your whole life routine. Now I'm feeling amazing and getting ready for the next race!

– Cecy Ae, Pennsylvania

"Staying Healthy and Injury-free"

I worked with Coach Shangrila initially with the Swim Bootcamp and saw my swim pace increase significantly over a short period of time. This occurred remotely with swim video feedback and 4/5x weekly swim workouts through Training Peaks. Swim Bootcamp also gave me access to the vast library of resources available on the Feisty Fox website, including drill videos, strength & mobility workouts, and yoga sessions.

This attention to detail led to me committing to a further five months of individual coaching to prepare me for a 70.3 triathlon. The personalized approach also helped me stay healthy and injury-free and helped me re-discover my running mojo. Thank you, Coach and Feisty Fox Family!

– John Wyatt, Arizona

"Achieving the Impossible With Training, Work & Family Balance"

I've always wanted to do a full Ironman race but never really thought it was possible. I did a 70.3 (half) about 8 years ago, and I thought that would be the pinnacle of my physical journey. Well, my wife encouraged me to sign up for a full 140.6 distance about a year ago, and I knew I couldn't complete it without some professional help. We looked into several training programs—some were in-person, some were virtual, and some were basically independent with just a basic plan to follow. We ultimately decided on Feisty Fox Coaching and would do it again in a heartbeat. The coaching pushed me hard enough to get it done but was also understanding regarding my busy schedule with work and family balance.

Here I am 3 weeks post-race with a smile on my face knowing that I finished something that few will ever even attempt—finishing happier and faster than I thought possible.

– Justin Wendzel, Business Owner, Michigan

"Back on Track"

I did the 30-day Swim Bootcamp. I had been off from swimming for a while, about 6 months. I wanted to kickstart my swimming again and regain some endurance and speed. Coach Shangrila really wants to help athletes improve and takes time discussing goals, roadblocks that may hinder them, and addressing them. I got a lot of feedback from my videos (although my videos were not the best quality lol) that was instrumental in me improving my technique. The camp is what I needed to get back on track. I am now getting coached for triathlon, and that is going very well too.

– Pamela Anne Coleman, Doctor, Texas

"From Fear of Swimming to Ironman"

2022 was the year my life changed for the BEST! Yes, 'BEST' ... A friend asked me to do a triathlon w/ her; mind you, this was after I just did a century bike ride around Lake Tahoe. I was winded and lacked oxygen, so naturally, I said 'Heck yeah! Let's do it! What's a triathlon?' ...

We signed up for the Lavaman Olympic ... 2 weeks prior to race day, March 16, 2020, the world shut down due to Covid. Friend said 'Hey! Let's swim at Aquatic Park ...' I was like 'Yes! Let's' ... so we went and THANK GOD the world shut down, because it turned out, I didn't know how to swim!!! I would have drowned on my first triathlon!!!!

Found a couple of coaches that helped me out in 2021 but not until 2022 when a friend recommended Coach Shangrila did I really learn how to swim. Not only did I learn, but I also was empowered to shed all anxieties, like the unknown lurking under water... of getting tired/getting a muscle cramp and then drowning... Months after the swim program, I was able to jump off a cliff and swim in the ocean without fear. I called Shangrila G. Rendon and Vineta G. Rendon the Swimmer Whisperers. They knew how to calm and empower my mind.

Bonus: After I learned how to correctly swim, I signed up to have Coach help me become a triathlete. BEST THING I've done in 2022 - 2023. Turned out, I wasn't cycling or running correctly either! I kept on getting injuries, and I've been cycling for 5 years prior!... *long story short, here I am, an Ironman. ONE YEAR later.*

It takes many people years to become Iron, but w/ Coach's guidance, and you're willing to work with her, YOU too can become an Ironman sooner than you think. I promise. I'm 57 years old ... if someone like me, who was out of shape, overweight, too lazy and too busy to do anything extra, can become Iron ... what more of a person who has the fire, the discipline and the drive?

Forever grateful, Coach, Shangrila G. Rendon!

– Sheila Alfaro, California

"Outstanding and Extremely In-Depth"

I highly recommend signing up for this training program. I recently completed the swimming boot camp, and the program is outstanding and extremely in-depth in regards to swimming technical aspects.

– Justin Wall, Lawyer, Indiana

"Equipped for the Future"

Coach Shangrila and her team helped me fine-tune my goals, come up with a customized plan, help me execute that plan, then tracked my results! Very helpful and tons of great guidance to make me faster while becoming more efficient in my swimming.

I highly recommend Feisty Fox Coaching—I did the swim bootcamp and saw the improvement I was hoping for. Plus, now I'm equipped to review and self-evaluate my stroke going forward to make sure I continue to improve—THANK YOU!

– Mark Birtch, Illinois

"Accomplished My Dream of 70.3 Injury-Free"

I am so very grateful to Feisty Fox Coaching, Coach Shangrila, Coach Claudia, and the rest of the team for helping me not only accomplish my dream of completing a 70.3 injury-free but also in becoming a stronger athlete both physically and mentally.

I highly recommend Feisty Fox Coaching. They have provided me with great coaching programs and have been flexible in adjusting training when I had limited time. Their coaching style is superb—great communication, feedback, and full of many resources to help one be their own best athlete. Great tribe too! What I admire most is their level of dedication and compassion they provide to each athlete. Best decision ever!

– Odette Oliveras, Florida

"Steady Improvements Every Week"

I cannot say enough good things about this coaching service! I stumbled upon the 'Ironman and Beyond' Facebook group. I joined the group in hopes to learn something about triathlons as I always have had a full Ironman on my list to conquer. I had already ordered a bike but I had never really rode competitively, on top of that I had never swam competitively either.

I took the plunge and signed up for the 'all in' service and never looked back! I have seen steady improvements week after week with all 3 disciplines! Looking back I don't know what I would've done without the guidance of Coach Shangrila and this group! The weekly improvements also build confidence! I would recommend this to anyone that is trying to achieve anything in the triathlon arena!

– Jeremy Dicken, Marathon Swimmer, IM Finisher and VP, Michigan

"From Average Age Grouper to World Championship"

Coach Shangrila and her team are just the best at teaching you everything you need to know about triathlon. Whether you are a newbie or an experienced age group athlete looking to achieve new goals Feisty Fox Coaching has a plan for you and a team to support you along the way.

I was able to go from an average age group athlete to qualifying for multiple Boston Marathons and the Ironman World Championship by improving all aspects of racing from mental mindset, nutrition, body maintenance, recovery and increasing my flexibility and mobility to stay injury free. I achieved so many goals and set new personal bests at every distance while also completing my first full distance Ironman events.

– Scott Steiner, Georgia

"Finally Seeing Improvement"

I have started and stopped many programs before but stuck with this one and finally saw an improvement in my swim times. This was due to the commitment FFC asks of you and you need to give. They are very supportive and want to see you improve. The video feedback on form is incredibly helpful.

– Karen George LeClair, 70.3 World Championship finisher, North Carolina

"From No Running to Achieving My 70.3 Goal"

Hi Coach Shangrila, I want to take a moment to thank you, I have learned so much from you, your humble desire to help others to live and become better is contagious.

Looking back in December 2022 before I started this program, with desires of improvement but not knowing how? The opportunity you offered me to help me and guide me to not settle to be average, gave me a goal, a challenge and fire up what I thought I couldn't do no more RUN due to my foot pain. Now I accomplish 70.3.

I experienced how great is this program and the 5 steps formula is amazing effective, and You, Vineta and all the Feisty Fox Coaching care not only for the sport but also for all the other areas of our lives that are important too, I HIGHLY RECOMMEND THIS PROGRAM.

– Carolina Robles, California

"From Zero to Success"

Thank you coach for all the wisdom and motivation! The best thing about the program is your ability to take someone with ZERO fitness, to someone that can achieve anything.

– Norman Romero, Business Owner, California

"Support Even When Unexpected Challenges Occurred"

I've followed Feisty Fox for a couple years, seeing everyone improve so much and be so supportive of each other. I finally decided to try the 30-day swim bootcamp.

I was not disappointed. During the personal phone calls with Shangrila and Vineta I got the support and advice that I needed. When I got sick they helped me work around it. When I got a twinge in my shoulder I immediately got advice on how to keep moving forwards. I am sure there is no challenge they can't meet.

I look forward to continuing my training with them to improve my entire tri training. Thanks so much for a great boot camp experience.

– Brad Rauh, South Carolina

"Unmatched Energy and Excitement"

The energy and excitement that Coach Shangrila and the team bring to the table is unmatched and just makes everything they do that much better.

From not just your training plan, but the video library, monthly calls, and live events on all topics around multi-sports make it even a better all-around program than just another training plan. While I may not be able to do everything, the choice is there for me and how much I want to dive in.

– Bob Woodruff, Sub 5:30 70.3 Finisher, Virginia

"A Life-Changing Community"

I am fairly new to triathlons and like most athletes. I found the swim to be the most challenging to train for. Especially if you don't know what good form and proper technique is supposed to feel like. I love the water, I am totally comfortable in the water, but I was struggling to learn how to swim competitively in a triathlon setting.

I found out quickly that a swimming is way more than just showing up to the pool or lake and just swim. I learned proper swim technique, what was wrong with my existing form and technique, proper drills to break bad habits, and how to incorporate those drills into my swim workouts.

Most importantly was the support of coach Shangrila, Coach Vineta, and the entire coaching staff. They were always responding quickly to any of my inquiries or needs. The swim feedback was quick and very descriptive. And all the resources available is a bonus... To see and feel my progress over the 30-days was incredible.

– Ron Vail, Engineer, New Hampshire

"Personalized and Supportive"

They personally know you and make custom workouts specific to your races. It is at your own time, and they also have classes, demos, and workouts you can access whenever. Supportive community too!

– Jackie Braun-McGee, Minnesota

"Nothing Less Than Incredible"

Feisty Fox Coaching provides an extremely comprehensive training program, and effective for even remote athletes. I was amazed at how effectively the coaches were able to help improve my technique and provide customized workouts based on my progress.

The program has an extensive array of resources to educate and motivate athletes. The best part were the online forums where we were able to share our successes and struggles. This like-minded community provides inspiration and camaraderie to help me excel in my goals.

I never knew what I was capable of, even though my coaches kept setting higher and higher goals. But with their coaching, I was able to swim faster, bike longer, and run without pain.

My experience has been nothing less than incredible as I would surprise myself week after week with the paces I would hit. This program has given me some of the most memorable experiences in my life, and I truly believe I would not have surpassed my goals without their help.

– Laura Lee, New Jersey

"Transformed My Life"

I wholeheartedly recommend Feisty Fox Coaching. Coach Shangrila and the team's unrelenting support, accountability, dedication, and guidance have transformed my life and my love for triathlon!! Feisty Fox is well worth the time and investment. Can't wait until next season... #RaceGoals

– Theresa E. Plaskett, New York

"Supportive And Encouraging"

I wanted to get better at swimming and stumbled across Feisty Fox 30-Day Swim Boot Camp. Coach Shangrila and Vineta and the other coaches made it a very supportive and encouraging experience. What Coach Shangrila didn't do was make it easy. Every week was a challenge. And I'm heading to Chattanooga 70.3 in May... look out swim! (Oh, Feisty Fox Coaching offered me more than just swim advice. The live body maintenance workouts and interviews with others who have achieved a lot in multi-sport were spot on too!)

– Tim Poole, Arkansas

"When you have a life outside of swim, bike, and run"

I came into Shangrila and her Feisty Fox training team a little skeptical. I have never really had any formal training in swimming (or any sport really) and was nervous to have someone analyze and correct what I was doing wrong (there was a lot).

The Feisty Fox crew is an understanding group, and Coach Shangrila's understanding of swim techniques is top-notch. She explains things and addresses issues with professionalism and extensive knowledge.

I mostly liked that she understands that us athletes do have a life outside of swim, bike, and run and does her best to work around your schedule but at the same time lets you know that the training must get done in order to succeed. Thank you, Shangrila and the team at Feisty Fox.

– Scott Chretien, Massachusetts

"Not Alone In My Fear"

The best decision I made was to reach out to Coach Shangrila and the Feisty Fox tribe to help reach my goals in my triathlon and then-some. Recovery from a year setback due to Covid and 7 weeks of terrible heel pain made me realize I needed help.

2 months of customized training, a great team of coaches instructing via Zoom, nutrition talks, bike care, daily body maintenance to heal my heel and avoid further injury... Sharing struggles and wins in the Feisty Fox tribe among other athletes made me feel part of a like-minded group. I was not alone in my fear of falling off my bike when going fast...

Training with intention is why the Feisty Fox Tribe works for me and will continue to help me to improve in my swim, bike, and run. I would not have placed 3rd in my age group had I tried training on my own.

– Zo Flores, Yoga & Aqua Aerobics instructor, CrossFit Trainer, Florida

"Superb"

Coach Shangrila and her coaching staff are amazing. I was looking for a coach to help prepare me for an upcoming Ironman triathlon and had reached out to several friends for recommendations and during that time Feisty Fox came across my news feed—I paused, listened, reached out, scheduled an information meeting, thought about it for a day, called Coach Shangrila back and here I am today better, stronger, wiser, confident, and excited!

No other coaching compares to what Feisty Fox offers. The level of resources and support provided is superb. The staff is professional, knowledgeable, and very accommodating. Programs are tailored to your lifestyle and adjustments are made to support your goals... I am blessed beyond measure to be part of the Feisty Fox family.

– Allyson Bennett, Pennsylvania

"From Stagnant to Swim Technique & Speed"

I signed up for the 30-Day Swim Boot Camp after watching several live videos of Coach Shangrila G. Rendon giving tips on how to improve on Ironman races and listening to her experience as an athlete herself. I did Swim Boot Camp to improve on my swim technique since I felt that I reached a stagnant point where I could no longer improve myself technique by going the self-taught method.

After 1 week of the boot camp, watching the practice videos that Coach provided, doing swim workouts, and taking the feedback from the swim analysis provided, I noticed a huge increase in swim technique. Going from a 2:30ish/min per 100 meters to 2:13/min per 100 meters. What really helped me was the swim analysis that were provided... I gained a lot from the 30-Day Swim Boot Camp... I'd recommend the 30-Day Swim Boot Camp to any athlete looking to improve their swim technique and pace.

– Carlos Eduardo Alvarez, Texas

"From Bodybuilder to Triathlete"

Joining Feisty Fox's coaching has been one of the best decisions ever made. As I embarked on the incredible journey to train for a triathlon, I realized I needed authentic guidance from professionals in a territory that was entirely new to me. Despite my 20 years of bodybuilding experience, diving into the world of triathlons was like stepping into uncharted waters.

With Coach Shangrila Rendon and her fantastic team by my side, I've found more than just a training program; I've discovered a community that believes in my potential. Their unwavering support, encouragement, and kindness have been a beacon of motivation through the challenges. The professionalism and expertise at Feisty Fox Coaching have empowered me to push my limits and grow in ways I never thought possible.

– Jorge Delgado, Colorado

"Sustainable Racing For Busy People"

I have had a dream of completing a 70.3 Ironman forever, but had no idea how to go about it. Then, I came across Feisty Fox Coaching...

I would highly recommend this amazing coaching team if you are considering sustainable racing. Their program feels built for busy people like me – it's all about smart and intentional training to fit in with your schedule, whatever that looks like, not just mindless hours. Plus, knowing your coach is a world-record holder like Shangrila Rendon is super inspiring!

They focus on preventing injuries, which is a huge deal for me, and they cover everything from swim technique to race strategy, and everything in between, to help you be successful in your goals. The Feisty Fox Coaching team are helping me build confidence and resilience in swimming, biking, and running to reach my triathlon goals without sacrificing my life in the process.

– Sarah Tribelhorn, California

Unstoppable:
The Smart
Training Method
For Busy Athletes

Achieving Triathlon Success Without Sacrificing
Life Balance or Getting Injured — For Triathletes,
Swimmers, Runners & Cyclists of All Levels

Shangrila Rendon

DISCLAIMER

The author of this book does not dispense medical, health, or sports performance advice but offers information of a general nature to support your fitness journey. This book is not intended to replace advice from qualified health professionals, coaches, or physicians. Always consult a medical or sports professional before beginning any new training program or making changes to your health and fitness regimen. Results may vary, and neither the publisher nor the author assumes liability for injuries, losses, or adverse outcomes that may occur as a result of using the methods or information described in this book. By using the information in this book, you accept full responsibility for your actions and outcomes.

Table Of Contents

Introduction: From Beginner to World-Class Coach

Hi, I'm Coach Shangrila, founder of Feisty Fox Coaching. We specialize in helping busy athletes of all levels maximize their health and achieve their biggest goals through triathlon and endurance sports.

Whether your goal is completing your first sprint triathlon, leveling up to cross the finish line at a 70.3 or full Ironman, conquering ultra swim/bike/run endurance races or qualifying for USAT Nationals, the Boston Marathon, or the 70.3 or full Ironman World Championship, we're here to help you crush it—even with limited time, past injuries, or the demands of a busy life.

The Journey to Helping Thousands

Over the last 20 years, I've helped thousands of athletes at all levels achieve their big goals—from finishing their first marathon, first sprint triathlon to completing their first Ironman, and even qualifying for the Ironman World Championship, USAT Nationals, or the Boston Marathon.

I've also guided athletes to success in ultra runs, cycling, marathon swimming, Ultraman, achieving podium finishes, and breaking personal records (PRs). But my journey didn't start there. In fact, it started with struggles much like yours.

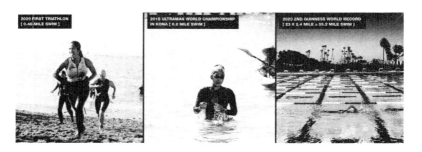

Before setting **two Guinness World Records**, completing 48 Ironman races (as of 2024), and competing in events like the Ironman World Championship in Kona, Ultraman World Championship, and Red Bull Trans Siberian Extreme—or even qualifying for the Boston Marathon and cycling across America—I could barely run for 15 minutes.

I couldn't ride with my shoes clipped to my bike, I barely knew how to swim, and I was terrified of deep water, let alone open-water swimming. Every time I raced, I was the last one out of the water.

Struggles and Challenges

I know what it's like to **struggle**, to feel like there's never enough time, and to battle the fear of failure. Alongside my sports journey, I was also completing my Master's degree in Engineering, climbing the corporate ladder, and dedicating 15 years to working full-time as an engineer and leader in medical device companies.

Personally, I faced and overcame significant **challenges**, including childhood abuse, alcohol addiction, sexual assault, an eating disorder, PTSD, severe depression, and suicidal ideation—emerging stronger from each. Balancing my engineering career, navigating my difficult past, training for triathlons and endurance races, spending time with family, friends and managing the demands of daily life certainly kept me busy.

But it also taught me the power of resilience, focus, and a systematic approach to achieving big goals.

Taking the Leap

Like many of you, I started out being very resourceful. I did all my own research, stayed independent, and worked hard to train the right way. I juggled time, signed up for weekend races to stay motivated, and kept pushing. But despite my efforts, I kept falling short. I felt disappointed. No matter how much I trained, it never felt like enough, and I wasn't reaching my full potential.

That's when I realized there had to be a better way—a smarter way.

I made a bold decision to leave my successful engineering career and fully immerse myself in mastering endurance sports. I quit my job, focused on yoga teacher training, and flew to Australia to dive deeply into swimming—a skill I had struggled with for years. There, I studied under world-class experts, analyzed elite swim techniques, and developed a comprehensive understanding of body movements across different body types and fitness levels. This transformative journey turned one of my greatest weaknesses into a strength.

But I didn't stop there. I worked as a spin instructor, honing my cycling knowledge while helping others achieve their fitness goals. I also traveled the world, competing in some of the most prestigious and extreme endurance races—not just to challenge myself but to test and refine the methods I was developing. These experiences pushed my body and mind to their limits, giving me invaluable insights into what works under the most grueling conditions.

Building the Smart Training Method

Over the years, I combined everything I learned to create a comprehensive and holistic approach to training:

- Completed triathlon coaching certifications

- Studied advanced swim techniques under world-class experts

- Certified in run gait analysis and coaching

- Attended cycling coaching courses, including cycling with power training

- Certified in TRX and strength training methods

- Completed yoga teacher training

- Gained knowledge in nutrition and physiology through targeted courses

- Completed injury prevention and management courses alongside medical professionals, with expertise in trigger point therapy, athlete assessments to identify root causes, and prescribing targeted exercises to proactively resolve issues.

Through years of trial and error and solving problems, I discovered what worked—and, more importantly, what didn't. I developed a system that transformed my life—not just as an athlete, but as a person.

This system didn't just help me overcome my fears of deep water, my struggles with time management, or my battles with injuries. It also taught me how to balance an incredibly busy life, recover from setbacks, and achieve more than I ever thought possible.

This journey wasn't just about gathering knowledge—I synthesized everything I learned into a **practical, results-driven approach** designed to empower athletes of all levels. Over time, this evolved into a comprehensive method I now call the **Smart Training Method.**

The Smart Training Method is a roadmap proven by science, real-world testing, and years of personal and professional experience. It's a comprehensive, balanced approach to triathlon and endurance sports training that prioritizes peak performance, injury prevention, and longevity while maintaining a fulfilling life outside of the sport. Whether you're just starting or chasing ambitious goals, this method works for athletes of all levels.

And the best part? This system isn't about training harder or longer—it's about **training smarter** and making the most of every minute you dedicate to your dreams.

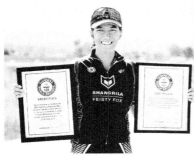
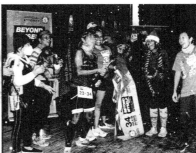

What is the Smart Training Method?

The Smart Training Method is based on five essential pillars—a framework that ensures a balanced and holistic approach to triathlon and endurance sports training. Each pillar plays a vital role in creating a system that prioritizes peak performance, injury prevention, longevity, and a fulfilling life outside the sport.

1. **Training -** Effective training is more than just putting in the hours. It's about structured, purposeful workouts tailored to your fitness level, goals, and schedule. Smart training maximizes progress by focusing on quality, not quantity—helping you improve while reducing the risk of overtraining.

2. **Nutrition -** Fueling your body isn't just about eating the right foods; it's about knowing what your body needs at different stages of training and recovery. Proper nutrition enhances performance, supports endurance, and accelerates recovery, ensuring you're always ready to perform at your best.

3. **Body Maintenance -** Injury prevention is the cornerstone of consistent training and long-term success. Regular body maintenance helps address imbalances, reduce strain, and keep you injury-free.

4. **Mental Fitness -** Your mindset is your greatest asset. Building mental resilience helps you overcome self-doubt, stay focused during challenging moments, and maintain discipline throughout your journey. Mental fitness ensures you're not just physically prepared but

emotionally and mentally equipped to succeed.

5. **Race Strategy** - Success on race day isn't just about being fit—it's about having a plan. From pacing and nutrition to handling transitions and race-day nerves, a solid race strategy ensures you execute your best performance when it matters most.

These pillars ensure a balanced and holistic approach, addressing all aspects of your performance, from workouts to mindset and recovery. This framework shifts the focus from "doing more" to **"doing what matters most."**

Smart Training for Busy Athletes: The Feisty Fox Way

At Feisty Fox Coaching, we understand that every athlete's journey is unique. That's why we don't believe in one-size-fits-all solutions. Our approach is built around the **Smart Training Method**, a proven framework that integrates **training, nutrition, body maintenance, mental fitness, and race strategy**. This comprehensive system helps athletes of all levels achieve their goals while staying balanced, injury-free, and fulfilled.

At the core of our Smart Training Method is the **360 Strategic Training framework**, which focuses on **four key components: Technique, Speed, Endurance, and Race Skills.** This purpose-driven approach ensures that every session aligns with your overall strategy, helping you build the skills and fitness you need while balancing effort and recovery.

Thousands of athletes—just like you—have followed this roadmap to achieve their triathlon and endurance sports dreams, all while staying injury-free and maintaining life balance. This system is built for busy athletes who face unique challenges:

- If you've never done a triathlon before
- If you're wanting to get back to running, cycling or swimming but don't know how
- If you're recovering from injuries or surgeries
- If you're balancing family, work, or frequent travel

- Had a long break from working out

- If you're a busy parent

- If you're over 40 and wondering if it's too late to start

This approach not only maximizes your progress but also minimizes burnout by balancing effort and recovery.

Together, the **Smart Training Method** and **360 Strategic Training** equip you with the tools to train effectively, maintain balance, and achieve your goals—whether it's completing your first sprint triathlon, crushing a 70.3, or conquering a full Ironman.

What You'll Get from This Book

This guide tackles the **three (3) most common challenges** faced by busy athletes:

"I Don't Have Enough Time to Train"

With a packed schedule, finding time to train can feel impossible. But the good news is, you don't need to spend 15-25 hours a week training to see results. This book shows you how to maximize your training by focusing on quality over quantity.

Through targeted, high-impact sessions and strategies to fit training into even the busiest schedule, you can achieve your goals in as little as 8-12 hours per week. Whether it's a lunch break swim, an early morning run, or a quick strength session, these methods will help you make time for what matters.

"I'm Afraid of Getting Injured"

Many athletes struggle with injuries that derail their progress and crush their confidence. Whether it's chronic pain, overuse injuries, or fear of re-injury, these setbacks can feel like roadblocks to your goals. This book introduces the **Smart Training Method**—a holistic framework that emphasizes proper training, injury prevention, nutrition, mindset and race strategy.

You'll learn how to listen to your body, build resilience, and avoid common mistakes that lead to injury. By following these steps, you'll stay injury-free and consistent in your training.

"I Don't Want to Sacrifice My Life Balance"

Balancing triathlon and endurance sports with work, family, and other responsibilities can feel overwhelming. Many athletes worry that pursuing their goals will come at the cost of their relationships or career. This guide will help you redefine what balance looks like.

Instead of trying to "do it all," you'll learn strategies to align your priorities, communicate with your loved ones, and involve them in your journey. You'll discover how to set boundaries, make time for what matters most, and enjoy the process—proving that it's possible to train for triathlon and endurance sports while living a full, balanced life.

By addressing these key challenges, this book provides not just solutions, but a roadmap for success. It's designed to inspire, guide, and empower you to pursue your triathlon and endurance sports dreams while staying injury-free, efficient, and balanced.

Inside, I'll walk you through the **Smart Training Method** and the **360 Strategic Training** framework, showing you how these systems integrate to create a plan that fits your life. You'll learn how to leverage all five pillars—**Training, Nutrition, Body Maintenance, Mental Fitness, and Race Strategy**—while ensuring every workout serves a purpose.

You'll also hear inspiring stories from athletes we've coached, including busy moms/dads high-achieving professionals, and retirees who thought their best days were behind them. Their journeys show what's possible when you train smarter, not harder.

How to Make the Most of This Book

This isn't just a book—it's your personalized guide to triathlon and endurance sports success. Here's how you can get the most out of this resource:

- **Utilize the Summaries and Actionable Steps:** At the end of each chapter, you'll find key takeaways and practical steps to implement immediately. Use these to create a clear roadmap for your training and stay focused on what truly matters.

- **Engage With Reflection Questions**: Throughout the book, you'll find thought-provoking questions designed to help you reflect on your training, mindset, and goals. Take the time to answer them honestly—you'll uncover valuable insights about where you are and where you want to go.

- **Free Training Resources:** If you'd like access to training resources, including stories from the athletes mentioned in this book, we have replays available. Scan the QR codes included in the book to get free access.

- **Reach Out for Support:** If you're inspired to go further or need additional guidance, email me at support@feistyfoxcoaching.com. I'm here to answer your questions, provide feedback, and help you take the next step in your triathlon and endurance sports journey.

This book is just the beginning. With the right tools, strategies, and support, your next big breakthrough is closer than you think. Let's make it happen together!

FREE GIFT: Bonus - Effective Time Management Worksheet for Athletes

I know how busy life can get when you're trying to balance training, work, and everything else. That's why I created the **Effective Time Management Worksheet for Athletes**—to help you train smarter, not harder.

It's super easy to use, and it'll make sure you stay on top of your game without feeling overwhelmed.

Here's how to grab it:

Just scan the QR code below or head to bit.ly/free-gifts-unstoppable.

As always, I've got your back. Let's crush those goals together!

ACCESS
FREE GIFTS

SCAN ME

What I Ask From You

This book was created to help you unlock your potential, and all I ask is:

1. **Read it with an open mind.** Whether you're new to endurance sports or a seasoned athlete, there's something here to help you reach the next level.

2. **Share your thoughts.** Let me know what resonated with you or what questions you have. Your feedback means the world to me!

3. **Pay it forward.** If you know someone who could benefit from this book, share it with them—it might just change their life.

Take Your Journey Even Further. Scan the QR Code Below to:

1. **Unlock exclusive Unstoppable book resources** to:

   a. Level up your swim, bike, run, and time management skills by applying the Smart Training Method and 360 Strategic Training tools from this book.

   b. Be inspired by real-life stories from athletes who overcame challenges, found solutions, and crushed their biggest goals.

   c. Dive deeper with step-by-step guidance through our coaching programs, tailored to help you implement these strategies into your life.

2. **Schedule a 15-minute Game Plan Call** to discuss your personal goals, identify the first steps to get you closer to achieving them and receive actionable advice tailored just for you.

Your best self - the strongest, healthiest and most empowered version of yourself is waiting. Let's get started.

RESERVE A
15 MIN
GAMEPLAN

SCAN ME

GET MORE
RESOURCES
SCAN ME

Chapter 1

I Don't Have Enough Time to Train

The key is not to prioritize what's on your schedule, but to schedule your priorities.

– Stephen Covey

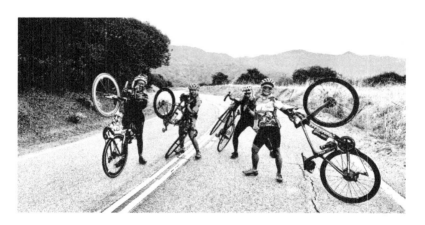

I remember the days when I was juggling a full-time engineering career, finishing my master's degree, studying for a run gait analysis certification, and training for my first triathlon.

Late nights, endless deadlines, and a packed schedule seemed like insurmountable obstacles.

There was no way I could train like the pros who had endless hours. But when I focused on making every minute count—like squeezing in swims during my lunch break or doing a 20-minute bike trainer session before work—things started to click.

It wasn't about doing more, it was about doing better. That shift not only helped me train smarter but gave me the confidence to chase my bigger dreams. If I could do it, you can too.

– Coach Shangrila

The Problem

Between work, family, and other responsibilities, time often feels like your most limited resource. For busy professionals, parents, and high achievers, squeezing triathlon and endurance sports training into an already packed schedule can seem impossible. The idea of devoting 15-25 hours a week to training may feel unrealistic and overwhelming.

But here's the truth: **you don't need endless hours to achieve your triathlon and endurance sports goals.** Success doesn't come from training longer—it comes from **training smarter,** whether you're preparing for a 70.3, a full Ironman, or just starting out in the sport.

The Solution: Time-Savvy Training

For busy professionals, parents, and high achievers, finding endless hours to train is simply not realistic. The Time-Savvy Training approach offers a solution that delivers results in as little as 8-12 hours per week.

By focusing on quality over quantity, this method ensures you achieve your goals without sacrificing your health, family, or work commitments. Here's how it works.

1. Prioritize Quality Sessions

Time is precious, so every workout should count. Instead of spending hours on long, unfocused sessions, Time-Savvy Training emphasizes high-impact workouts that produce measurable improvements.

- **Build Endurance**: Incorporate specific sessions that gradually enhance stamina without overtraining.

- **Improve Technique**: Focused technique drills and skills-based exercises not only make you more efficient but also conserve energy on race day.

- **Develop Strength**: Short 5-20 mins targeted body maintenance & strength workouts build resilience, prevent injuries, and enhance performance across all three disciplines.

- **Be Purposeful**: Understand the goal of each workout—why you're doing it and how it contributes to your progress. This eliminates the "just checking the box" mentality and replaces it with intentional, results-driven training.

For instance, instead of running 10 miles slowly and unfocused, a targeted interval session with speed and hill work can deliver better results in less time.

2. Plan Around Your Life

Triathlon training should fit into your lifestyle—not the other way around. Time Savvy Training is designed to work with your schedule and priorities.

- **Identify Quiet Times**: Early mornings, lunch breaks, or late evenings can be ideal windows for training. For example, a 30-minute swim before work or a quick run while the kids are at soccer practice can make a big difference.

- **Incorporate Family Time**: Training doesn't have to take you away from your loved ones. Ride your bike on a trainer while watching a family movie or invite your kids to join you for a post-run stretching session. Not only do you train, but you also set an example of healthy living.

- **Stay Flexible**: Life is unpredictable, so having a flexible plan allows you to adapt without losing momentum.

Athletes like Gwen, a full-time physical therapist, mom of five, followed this principle. She scheduled just 5-6 days of training per week, with one being a complete rest day for the family. With proper planning and communication, she trained consistently and achieved her first full Ironman in 6 months.

3. Use Efficient Training Blocks

Maximizing time isn't just about cramming workouts into your day—it's about structuring them strategically. Efficient training blocks are key to achieving the most progress in the least amount of time.

- **Combine Sessions**: Brick workouts (e.g., bike + run) are perfect for triathletes, simulating race conditions while cutting down training hours. For example, a 90-minute bike ride followed by a 20-minute run can prepare you for transitions without requiring separate sessions.

- **Target Key Skills**: Each block should focus on building one or more critical race-day components—endurance, speed, technique or race-skills. For instance, pairing a swim session with strength training saves time while addressing complementary needs.

- **Maximize Recovery**: Short, intense blocks allow more time for recovery, preventing burnout and ensuring every session is productive.

Take Reggie, a business owner, husband, and father of three who often travels for work. By using efficient training blocks and a clear plan, he completed his first full Ironman in under 14 hours without injury—all while maintaining his family and work commitments.

Why This Approach Works

Time Savvy Training shifts the focus from doing more to training with intentions. It's not about endless hours; it's about maximizing every minute of effort. Whether you're new to triathlon or training for a 70.3 or full Ironman, this method equips you to succeed within the time you have.

By implementing these principles, you'll train smarter, achieve more, and maintain a balanced life—all while preparing for your best race performance.

Quality Over Quantity: Training Smarter, Not Longer

Training volume plays a role in any well-rounded plan, but it's not the ultimate goal. Long hours of training contribute to endurance, but there's no single magic number of hours that guarantees success. Instead, success hinges on the quality of your efforts and how well you integrate all aspects of your training.

Focusing solely on one pillar—**Training**—without addressing the others in the **Smart Training Method** can undermine your results. For example:

- **Nutrition:** Even the most structured interval workout won't achieve its purpose if your body isn't properly fueled. Neglecting to eat adequately before and after a session can lead to subpar performance, poor recovery, and stagnation.

- **Body Maintenance:** Skipping regular mobility and strength exercises increases the risk of muscle imbalances, tightness, or weakness. These issues not only limit your ability to hit high-quality efforts during workouts but can also lead to injury over time.

- **Mindset:** A distracted mind or lack of focus during training diminishes the effectiveness of a workout. Without practicing body awareness, you may execute exercises incorrectly or miss the opportunity to push yourself to your full potential. Mental fitness ensures that you're fully engaged and purposeful in every session.

A high-quality training session doesn't just mean completing the workout—it means completing it with purpose, focus, and under the best possible conditions to maximize its benefit. By addressing **all five (5) pillars—Training, Nutrition, Body Maintenance, Mindset, and Race Strategy**—you ensure your sessions contribute to sustainable progress.

Hours Trained vs. Benefits Gained

This simple chart below illustrates a key truth about training: more isn't always better. When 80% of your training is **focused and intentional**, you'll achieve 100% of your progress. But the remaining 20%—unfocused, low-quality sessions—can lead to diminishing returns

80% Focused Quality Training = 100% Progress

The **light portion** of the pie chart (80%) represents the time spent on purposeful, high-impact workouts. These are sessions with a specific goal: improving strength, speed, endurance, or technique. When training is intentional, focused, and aligned with your goals, you maximize results with less time.

- **Examples of Quality Training:**

  - High-intensity interval sessions (HIIT) for cardiovascular gains.

  - Tempo runs to improve your lactate threshold.

  - Structured recovery sessions to allow for proper adaptation.

20% Unfocused Volume = Diminishing Returns

The **dark portion** (20%) highlights time spent on unfocused, low-quality training. This includes:

- Logging junk miles without a specific purpose.

- Training excessively without clear goals or a recovery strategy.

While you may feel like you're working harder, these sessions contribute little to your progress and increase the risk of burnout and injury.

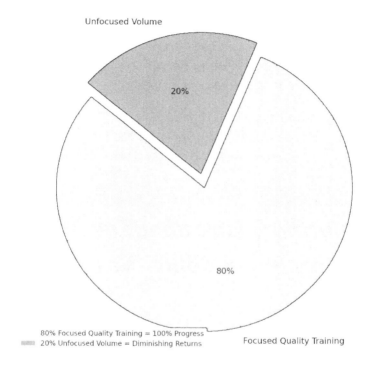

Unfocused Volume

20%

80%

80% Focused Quality Training = 100% Progress
20% Unfocused Volume = Diminishing Returns

Focused Quality Training

The Takeaway: Train Smarter, Not Harder

- More training hours do not always equal better results.

- **Focused, intentional sessions** bring the biggest return on your time and energy investment.

Chris Bailey, productivity expert and author of The Productivity Project, reminds us that true efficiency comes from prioritizing what truly matters, not just filling our time with activity. As he puts it:

"Productivity isn't about doing more; it's about doing the right things."

This principle is key to training smarter. Triathlon success isn't about how many hours you spend swimming, cycling, or running—it's about ensuring every session serves a specific purpose. By focusing on workouts that align with your goals, you make the most of your limited time and energy while seeing measurable results.

What Science Says About Training Smarter

Athletes often assume that success comes from piling on training hours. However, research and evidence consistently show that **focused, high-quality sessions** deliver greater results than sheer volume.

A study conducted at **McMaster University** found that **high-intensity interval training (HIIT)** can produce the same endurance and cardiovascular benefits as longer, moderate-intensity workouts—**but in significantly less time**. In the study, just **10 minutes of HIIT**—including one minute of intense effort—was as effective as a 50-minute steady-state endurance session (Burgomaster et al., 2008).

This research is a game-changer for time-crunched athletes. It proves that even with limited hours, you can achieve your triathlon goals by training with purpose and intensity. A 60-minute interval session or tempo run, for example, can provide the physiological adaptations needed to build endurance, speed, and fitness without overwhelming your schedule.

Additionally, elite coaches like Steve Magness, in The Science of Running, emphasize that the body adapts to **specific stress**, not just time spent training. This means that every session must have a clear objective—whether it's increasing your lactate threshold, building strength, or improving technique. "It's not about how many hours you put in," he explains, "but what you put into those hours."

The bottom line? Training smarter—focusing on quality, not quantity—allows you to progress faster while balancing work, family, and life. By choosing **high-impact workouts** that align with your goals, you'll see greater results in less time.

How the Pros Train Smarter: Insights from Elite Athletes

Even the world's best athletes don't rely on endless hours of training to succeed. They optimize every session, focus on purposeful recovery, and manage their time efficiently. Here's how top performers and coaches approach quality over quantity:

Chrissie Wellington (4x Ironman World Champion)

1. Despite balancing her training with commitments as an activist and author, Chrissie prioritized key sessions and ensured each one counted.

2. In her book A Life Without Limits, she emphasizes quality over volume: "It's not about the number of hours you train; it's about making every session count."

Jan Frodeno (Olympic Gold Medalist & Ironman World Champion)

1. Jan's coach emphasizes a polarized training model—80% of sessions are low-intensity, and 20% are high-intensity. This ensures maximum gains without burnout.

2. "It's not about how many hours you put in but what you put into those hours."

Eliud Kipchoge (Marathon World Record Holder)

1. Kipchoge trains in a minimalist camp environment, optimizing his schedule for quality workouts and deliberate recovery.

2. He believes discipline and focus are the foundations of success: "Only the disciplined ones in life are free. If you are undisciplined, you are a slave to your moods and your passions."

Time, Energy & Attention: The Keys to Unlocking Productivity in Triathlon and Endurance Sports Training

Success in triathlon and endurance sports—or any significant goal—isn't just about the number of hours you dedicate. It's about how efficiently you manage your **time, energy, and attention.**

These three resources are intricately connected, and when balanced, they enable you to reach peak performance.

Whether you're navigating a demanding career, family responsibilities, or personal challenges, understanding and leveraging these elements can transform both your training and your life.

Take Jeremy, for example. Within just eight months, he trained for and completed a 70.3 triathlon, a century ride, an 8.2-mile marathon swim around Mackinac Island, and his second full Ironman at Chattanooga. As a VP in his company, a husband, and a father actively involved in his daughter's track meets and school activities, Jeremy excelled by mastering his time, energy, and attention. His success wasn't about doing it all—it was about doing the right things well.

Jeremy's approach was simple yet profound: he was 100% committed to his goal, ensuring that his workouts got done no matter what. He gave full focus to work, family, and training by setting clear boundaries and prioritizing what mattered most in each area of his life.

His key strategy? Sleeping early to wake up refreshed for focused, efficient training sessions before the day's demands began. By aligning his actions with his priorities, Jeremy not only achieved his athletic goals but also maintained a balanced and fulfilling life.

The Three Pillars of Productivity in Training

1. **Time** is the foundation of your day. The way you structure your schedule determines how much you can achieve.

2. **Energy** fuels your ability to carry out tasks. Physical and mental stamina play a key role in how well you execute your plan.

3. **Attention** ensures you're fully engaged and focused on what matters most, minimizing wasted effort.

When any one of these pillars is neglected, your productivity suffers. By mastering these pillars, you can align your resources with your goals and create momentum in your training.

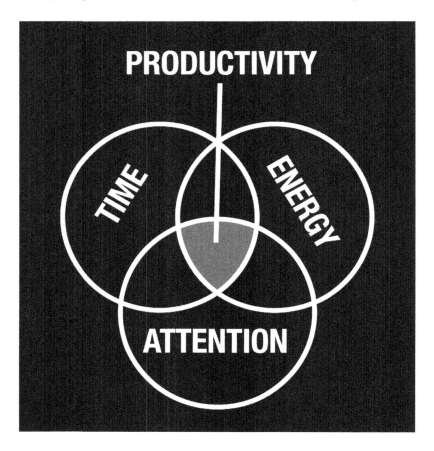

Rest as a Productivity Multiplier

Getting enough sleep is critical for athletes. It's during sleep that your body repairs itself and your mind recovers, preparing you for the demands of the day ahead.

For triathletes, sleep isn't just about rest; it's a vital part of recovery. Without it, your energy reserves deplete faster, and your focus wanes, resulting in inefficient training. Jeremy prioritized early bedtimes to ensure his training sessions were productive and his family commitments were met.

Sleep directly impacts your ability to complete workouts efficiently and reduces the likelihood of injury. When you're well-rested, you approach each training session with the energy and attention needed to maximize its benefits.

Mindset: The Often Overlooked Pillar of Success

Your mindset is as crucial to your success as your physical preparation. No matter how meticulously crafted your training plan is, if you're distracted, mentally scattered, or harboring self-doubt, you won't reach your full potential. A focused and purposeful mindset enables you to stay present, push through challenges, and maximize every session.

Take Erik, for example. As a father of four and a business owner, Erik's time was limited, but his mindset set him apart. When Erik trained, he gave 100% of his focus and attention to the task at hand, whether it was an endurance ride, a speed session, or a recovery swim. This unwavering focus helped him qualify for the Ironman World Championship in Kona with a personal best of 11:05:19, just in his second full Ironman. He also achieved a remarkable 70.3 PR of 5:02:00, demonstrating how a focused mindset can translate into exceptional results.

Erik's success wasn't just about physical effort—it was about mental clarity. He approached each session with a clear purpose, understanding that every minute spent training mattered. This mindset didn't just allow him to meet his goals; it enabled him to exceed them.

Practicing mindfulness and body awareness during workouts is another critical component of a strong mindset. For example, instead of just completing laps during a swim, focus on stroke efficiency, breathing rhythm, and body position. Similarly, on a long ride, tune into how your body feels and adjust your posture or cadence as needed. These small, intentional adjustments, driven by focused attention, compound over time to deliver significant improvements.

Erik's story is proof that cultivating a strong, focused mindset can elevate your training from good to extraordinary. It's not just about the hours you put in; it's about the quality of your attention during those hours. When you show up with purpose and clarity, success becomes inevitable.

The Interconnection of Time, Energy, and Attention

Imagine starting a swim session after a sleepless night, distracted by work emails, and without a clear goal. The session is likely to be frustrating and unproductive. Contrast that with a session where you're well-rested, focused, and intentional. This stark difference underscores how interconnected time, energy, and attention are in determining your success.

By prioritizing rest, eliminating distractions, and approaching each session with clarity, you can achieve more in less time. This integrated approach ensures that your efforts align with your goals, creating a cycle of productivity that fuels both your training and your life.

Apply the Framework to Your Life

How can you start applying these principles today?

Begin by assessing your current habits:

- Are you getting enough rest?

- Are you allowing distractions to dilute your focus?

- Are you setting clear goals for each session?

Use Gwen, Reggie, Jeremy and Erik's stories as a reminder that with the right mindset and approach, even the busiest schedules can accommodate ambitious goals.

Take control of your time, energy, and attention, and watch your triathlon journey—and life—transform.

Chapter 1 Summary: "I Don't Have Enough Time to Train"

Key Insight: You don't need endless hours to train for a triathlon. Success comes from training smarter, not longer, and integrating triathlon training into your busy life.

Core Strategies:

1. **Focus on Quality Over Quantity**: Every session should have a clear purpose—build endurance, refine technique, or develop strength.

2. **Integrate Training Into Your Life**: Look for windows of opportunity like early mornings, lunch breaks, or family-friendly training options.

3. **Use Efficient Workouts**: Combine sessions, like a bike-run brick, or pair strength training with a short swim to maximize progress in less time.

4. **Align Time, Energy, and Attention**: Ensure your priorities and resources match your goals, and prioritize rest and recovery.

Real-Life Inspiration: Athletes like Gwen, Reggie, Jeremy and Erik proved that even with demanding schedules, consistency and purposeful effort can lead to success.

Actionable Steps

Here are five steps you can take this week to start managing your time and training smarter:

1. **Analyze Your Schedule**: Look for 20-30 minute gaps in your day and plan focused workouts during those times.

2. **Plan One Quality Session**: Choose one session to focus on a specific goal, like improving swim technique or running intervals, instead of just "checking a box."

3. **Combine Workouts**: Replace two separate sessions with a brick workout, like a 60-minute bike followed by a 15-minute run.

4. **Communicate with Your Family**: Share your goals and find ways to include them—such as stretching together or training during family activities.

5. **Prioritize Sleep**: Start going to bed 30 minutes earlier to ensure you're rested and ready to train efficiently.

Reflection Questions

End the chapter by reflecting on how to apply what you've learned:

- What's one step you can take this week to fit training into your schedule?

- How can you maximize the quality of your workouts?

- Who can you involve in your training journey to help you stay motivated?

Chapter 2

Stay Injury Free - Training Smarter, Not Harder

Don't train in pain—your body knows what it needs. Pay attention, and it will show you the way.

– Shangrila Rendon

I'll never forget the time I ignored the warning signs my body was giving me.

I was training for one of my marathon races, and I pushed through a nagging pain in my knee, convincing myself it would go away.

I even told myself, 'No pain, no gain. I've got this.' But instead of getting better, it got worse. Eventually, I couldn't even run without limping.

That setback cost me weeks of training, but more than that, it drained my energy and crushed my confidence. For a while, I wasn't just an injured athlete—I wasn't a happy one either.

That experience taught me one of the most valuable lessons as an athlete: pain isn't something to 'power through.' It's your body's way of asking for help.

Now, I remind my athletes—and myself—that smart training means respecting what your body is telling you. When you listen to it, you avoid setbacks and come back stronger

Don't train in pain—it's never worth the risk.

– Coach Shangrila

One of the biggest fears holding people back from training for triathlons is the **fear of getting injured**.

This fear isn't unfounded—many injuries stem from overtraining, poor technique, or a lack of structured guidance. However, the good news is that injuries are preventable with the right approach, one that prioritizes balance, structure, and long-term health over sheer intensity or volume.

A study by **Meeusen et al. (2013)** highlights the risks of overtraining syndrome and emphasizes the importance of balancing training load with adequate recovery. The research found that structured recovery periods and varied intensity levels not only reduced injury risk but also improved athletic performance over time. Overtraining, on the other hand, led to fatigue, performance decline, and increased risk of injury.

Training Stress vs. Recovery Balance

The graph highlights the difference between balanced training with proper recovery and unbalanced stress leading to injury risk.

- **Unbalanced Training Stress (Dark dotted)**: Shows a steep rise in training load without adequate recovery, surpassing the **Injury Threshold**.

- **Balanced Training Stress (Light solid)**: Demonstrates a sustainable increase in training load with planned recovery.

- **Balanced Recovery (Dark solid)**: Recovery is increased alongside training, ensuring steady performance gains.

- **Unbalanced Recovery (Light dotted)**: A decline in recovery results in stagnation or regression.

Athletes who balance training stress and recovery maintain progress, avoid injuries, and perform consistently over time.

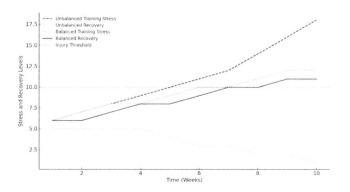

Why Do Injuries Happen?

Most injuries aren't the result of one big mistake; they're the culmination of small issues that build up over time. Common culprits include:

- Running, swimming or cycling with poor technique

- Ignoring signs of fatigue

- Doing too much too soon

- Skipping essential body maintenance or injury prevention routines

This is why structured training is so important—it helps you build strength and endurance gradually while addressing the areas that need the most attention.

At Feisty Fox Coaching, we believe in the principle: **Don't train in pain.** Pain is a signal, and ignoring it can lead to long-term setbacks. Open communication between athletes and coaches is vital.

Athletes like Zo, a yoga instructor and CrossFit trainer, show that injuries often require more than isolated fixes like stretching or massage. Her heel pain persisted for weeks until she adopted a comprehensive plan that included refining technique, addressing daily activities, and balancing training stress with recovery. Through this approach, she not only healed but returned stronger and injury-free.

Discomfort may signal fatigue or tightness, while persistent or sharp pain often indicates a weak link that could lead to injury or impact race-day performance. If pain arises during training, consider how it might escalate during a high-stress race.

Addressing root causes early is critical to maintaining injury-free, consistent training.

The Smart Training Method

Our injury-prevention and performance system isn't about training harder—it's about training smarter. The **5 Pillars of the Feisty Fox Smart Training Method** ensure a holistic, injury-free approach:

1. **Training**: Structured workouts tailored to your level, goals, and schedule, improving performance while reducing overtraining risks.

2. **Nutrition**: Proper fueling and hydration to support recovery, energy, and endurance.

3. **Body Maintenance**: Regular exercises and routines to strengthen weak areas, correct imbalances, and recover fast.

4. **Mental Fitness**: A strong, focused and positive mindset to stay disciplined and resilient through challenges.

5. **Race Strategy**: Detailed plans for pacing, nutrition, transitions, and energy management to optimize race-day performance.

These pillars work together to create a balanced, sustainable system that prepares you not just for one race but for long-term success in triathlon and endurance sports.

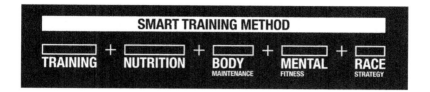

FREE GIFT: Bonus - Smart Training Method Worksheet

Training smarter doesn't mean doing it all by yourself. That's why I'm sharing the **Smart Training Method Worksheet**—a simple, step-by-step guide to help you find and fix gaps in your training.

This worksheet will help you:

- Spot what's working and what's not.

- Build a plan that keeps you consistent.

- Show up on race day confident and ready to perform!

How to Get It:

Just scan the QR code below or go to bit.ly/free-gifts-unstoppable.

You're one step closer to smarter training and stronger results. You've got this!

SCAN ME

ACCESS
FREE GIFTS

Introducing 360 Strategic Training

While the Feisty Fox Smart Training Method provides the foundational pillars for injury-free and balanced triathlon preparation, **360 Strategic Training** takes it a step further. It dives into the **what, why, and how** of the technical components of triathlon success. Also, it's a focused system designed to integrate **Technique, Speed, Endurance, and Race Skills** into your training. These four components ensure that every part of your preparation is optimized, helping you achieve a strong, efficient, and confident race day performance without overtraining.

Many athletes fall into the trap of simply covering distances to "check the box," but distance alone isn't enough. Without attention to key aspects like efficiency, pacing, and race-specific readiness, you may end up overworking your body or feeling underprepared on race day. That's where 360 Strategic Training transforms the way you train.

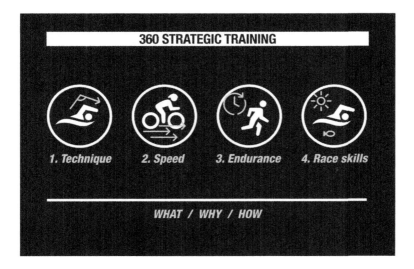

Technique: The Foundation of Efficiency

Technique is the backbone of triathlon success. Whether it's perfecting your swim stroke, dialing in your bike cadence, or improving your running posture, refining technique ensures that every movement is efficient and effective. Good technique helps conserve energy, avoid injury, and make training at higher intensities more productive.

The Swimming Trap: When Practice Doesn't Make Perfect

I asked an athlete, "Are you working on your swim technique?" They confidently replied, "Yes, I wear fins, use paddles, and watch YouTube videos for technique drills."

"That's great," I said. "But how do you know if you're doing the swim technique correctly?" They paused and admitted, "Uh, I don't know."

This is where many athletes go wrong. Practicing drills and using tools like paddles and fins is helpful, but if you're practicing improper technique, you're reinforcing bad habits. Worse, you can build a false sense of confidence, believing you're improving when you're actually ingraining inefficiencies or even setting yourself up for injury.

Improving swim technique isn't just about knowing what needs to be corrected—it's about learning **how** to make those corrections, confirming you are indeed executing proper technique, understanding your body movements in the water and consistently practicing the right habits. It's not a one-and-done process; it requires dedication, feedback, and the patience to implement small but critical changes over time.

As a freestyle swim technique expert, I've seen firsthand what works for athletes. Constant feedback is essential—whether from a coach or through video analysis. Tracking progress, especially pace improvements, helps ensure the changes are taking effect. Understanding where the athlete is coming from—their prior experience, limitations, and current skill level—provides a foundation for building the right adjustments.

Consistency is also key. Showing up regularly to the pool and dedicating time to focused practice creates lasting habits. Body awareness plays a crucial role as well; athletes need to feel their movements and share what they experience. This open feedback loop allows us to fine-tune techniques together, ensuring they're always moving closer to mastery.

With the right approach, swimming doesn't just improve—it transforms into a powerful, energy-efficient discipline that carries over to the rest of the race.

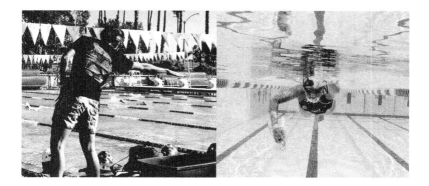

Running Smarter, Not Harder

When many athletes start running, they think all it takes is tying their shoes and hitting the pavement. I used to think the same—believing that sheer effort alone would be enough to succeed. But as I've evolved as a coach and become a certified run gait analyst, I've learned that proper running technique isn't just helpful—it's a game-changer.

Technique matters in every aspect of running. It's not just about improving performance; it's about reducing unnecessary strain, conserving energy, and protecting your body from injuries. Whether tackling the marathon leg of a full Ironman, the half marathon of a 70.3, or chasing a Boston Marathon qualifying time, refining technique becomes crucial—especially as fatigue sets in.

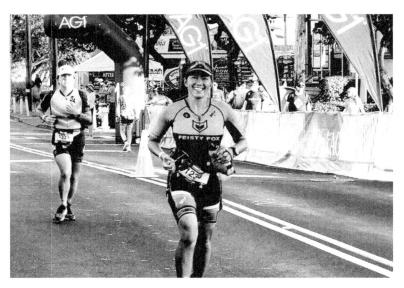

I've worked with athletes to identify and correct inefficiencies in their form, from posture to stride mechanics. These adjustments can lead to remarkable transformations. I've seen athletes eliminate recurring hip and knee pain, reduce blisters, and even achieve PRs by simply focusing on technique. One athlete told me, "Coach, I wasn't even putting in more effort, but my legs felt great, and I ran a PR!"

Personally, I've experienced this too. Even in my own races, I remain mindful of my form from the starting line to the finish, especially during the final, most grueling miles. By maintaining proper posture and efficient strides, I've improved not only my own performance but also my recovery and long-term running sustainability. My goal as a coach is to pass these lessons on—so every athlete can run smarter, not harder.

Cycling: Beyond Pedaling Hard

I've seen many athletes start out thinking cycling is all about brute strength—pedaling as hard as possible to get from point A to point B. This mindset often overlooks the critical role of technique in unlocking true performance potential.

Proper cycling isn't just about power; it's about efficiency. Many athletes don't realize that the right gearing, cadence, and pedaling technique not only increase power output but also improve run performance and reduce the risk of injury. Poor technique doesn't just slow you down; it wastes energy, creates unnecessary strain on the body, and can lead to long-term wear and tear.

When I began refining technique with athletes, everything changed. Engaging the right muscle groups, maintaining optimal cadence, and applying power efficiently transformed their rides. These improvements didn't just make them faster on the bike—they also saved energy for the run and enhanced their overall race performance.

For example, learning how and when to shift gears ensures you're not overloading your muscles unnecessarily. Understanding seated versus standing power dynamics helps adapt to different terrains, while honing pedal stroke efficiency ensures you're maximizing every revolution without losing energy.

The results I've seen from these adjustments have been remarkable. Athletes often tell me they feel stronger, more confident, and less fatigued after implementing these techniques. Some even report that their newfound efficiency on the bike carries over to unexpected gains in their running, allowing for stronger finishes and better race-day outcomes.

Cycling isn't just about pedaling hard—it's about pedaling smart. With the right approach, you can ride faster, conserve energy, and set yourself up for success in every aspect of your race.

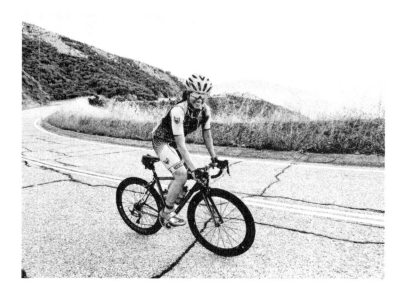

Speed and Pacing: The Art of Balancing Intensity

To develop speed and endurance effectively, each workout must have a clear objective—whether it's building speed, enhancing aerobic capacity, or promoting recovery. Speed is developed through targeted high-intensity efforts, while pacing ensures that speed is sustainable over long distances.

Athletes often mistake training hard in every session for progress, but this approach can lead to overtraining, fatigue, and even injury. Instead, elite performance is achieved by balancing high- and low-intensity efforts, as shown in the Elite Intensity graph. This polarized approach alternates between intense, purposeful sessions and low-intensity recovery, creating the perfect formula for maximizing performance while allowing for adequate recovery.

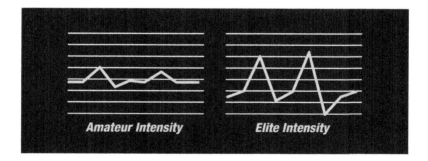

The Role of Metrics in Speed and Pacing

To measure and refine intensity, tracking key metrics is essential for building speed, maintaining pacing, and optimizing performance. Athletes can benefit from evaluating:

- **Heart Rate:** A vital metric for assessing aerobic efficiency, tracking effort levels, and monitoring recovery capacity. It ensures you're training within the right zones for endurance and performance gains.

- **RPE (Rate of Perceived Exertion):** A subjective yet powerful tool for gauging effort. It helps athletes fine-tune their training intensity, even without access to advanced devices.

- **Pace/Speed:** Crucial for measuring consistency, managing effort across distances, and achieving race-day targets in swimming, cycling, and running.

- **Power Output:** Particularly for cycling, power provides a direct measure of intensity, ensuring targeted efforts that build strength and endurance efficiently.

- **Cadence:** Key for optimizing rhythm and efficiency in cycling and running. A well-balanced cadence reduces fatigue and improves overall movement economy.

- **Stroke Rate:** Specifically for swimming, stroke rate helps monitor efficiency and rhythm in the water. Balancing stroke rate with distance per stroke ensures maximum propulsion without wasted energy.

Regularly monitoring these metrics helps athletes fine-tune their intensity and ensures every session has a purpose.

Why Pacing Matters

Athletes often overestimate the value of all-out effort in every session. While pushing hard has its place, consistently training at high intensities can lead to overtraining, fatigue, or injury. Pacing is about strategic effort—knowing when to push and when to hold back.

A practical approach to pacing includes:

- **High-Intensity Sessions:** Focus on intervals, hill repeats, or threshold efforts to push limits.

- **Low-Intensity Recovery Sessions:** Promote adaptations without overtaxing the body, ensuring sustainable progress.

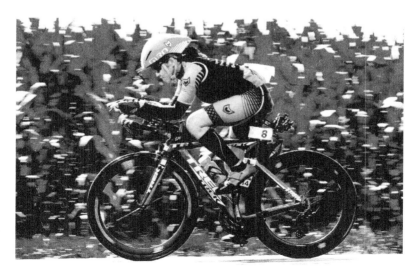

Integrating Speed into 360 Strategic Training

Speed development is a cornerstone of 360 Strategic Training, alongside technique, endurance, and race-specific skills. This comprehensive approach ensures athletes achieve balanced growth without risking burnout. Here's how speed is developed within this framework:

- **Technique First:** Efficient form reduces energy waste and allows for faster speeds at lower effort.

- **Smart Progression:** Gradually increasing intensity and duration to build resilience without burnout.

- **Recovery Focus:** Using low-intensity sessions to consolidate gains and prepare for the next high-effort workout.

Why Balance is Key

Training isn't just about going hard; it's about knowing when to recover. High-intensity efforts stress your body, but without adequate low-intensity recovery, those stresses can accumulate and hinder progress. A well-designed program integrates periods of peak effort with adequate recovery, creating a rhythm that mirrors the Elite Intensity graph.

A Personalized Approach for Real Results

At Feisty Fox Coaching, we emphasize a personalized, adaptable system that combines data and communication. Metrics like heart rate, RPE, pacing, power, cadence, and stroke rate allow us to refine each athlete's plan in real-time, ensuring training aligns with their current state and goals.

Our approach considers the full picture of an athlete's life, including:

- How their body feels during and after workouts.

- Unexpected challenges like poor sleep, long workdays, or elevated stress.

- Adjustments needed to balance training, work, and family demands.

This personalized methodology ensures training complements your life, not competes with it, and fosters sustainable progress.

Why This Matters

The goal isn't just to improve performance—it's to help athletes thrive holistically. Training should enhance, not overshadow, your life. By focusing on balance, recovery, and personalized strategies, you can achieve your goals injury-free while maintaining alignment with your personal and professional life.

Endurance: Building Long-Lasting Strength and Durability

Endurance training goes beyond adding distance—it's about creating a foundation for sustainable athletic success while balancing intensity, recovery, and cumulative stress. As a core pillar of the 360 Strategic Training framework, endurance focuses on developing the stamina, durability, and resilience required for triathlon and long-term fitness.

The Role of Zone 2 in Endurance Training

Zone 2, the aerobic heart rate zone, is essential for effective endurance training. It's the intensity level where your body efficiently burns fat for fuel, characterized by a conversational pace that feels sustainable. However, many athletes inadvertently train at higher intensities during their Zone 2 sessions, slipping into a "grey area" that undermines endurance development.

True Zone 2 training requires precision, guided by pacing, heart rate, RPE and threshold data. Staying within this zone enhances cardiovascular efficiency while minimizing fatigue, laying the groundwork for both endurance and recovery.

Beyond Distance: Balancing Intensity and Stress Across Sports

Building endurance isn't just about increasing mileage; it involves balancing volume, intensity, and stress across the swim, bike, and run disciplines. Key considerations include:

- **Intensity Management:** Ensuring that endurance sessions maintain proper intensity, particularly in Zone 2, to maximize aerobic gains and minimize unnecessary fatigue.

- **Cumulative Stress:** Accounting for the overall training load from all three sports, along with external stressors, to allow for proper recovery and adaptation.

- **Strategic Progression:** Gradual increases in distance or duration should be paired with controlled intensity to support long-term development without overloading the body.

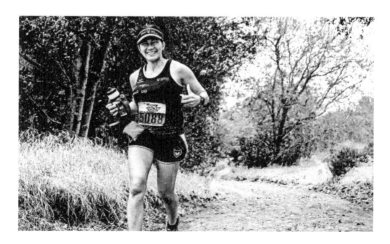

Nutrition and Recovery: Supporting Endurance Training

Endurance training places significant demands on your body, making nutrition and recovery essential to success:

- **Nutrition:** Proper fueling before, during, and after sessions ensures sustained energy and aids recovery. Training your gut for race-day nutrition is an integral part of long-distance preparation.

- **Body Maintenance:** Practices such as foam rolling, mobility exercises, and targeted strength training enhance durability and reduce injury risk, ensuring your body is equipped to handle increased endurance demands.

Building Long-Term Durability

The true goal of endurance training is to develop long-term durability—the ability to perform consistently and injury-free over years, not just one race. This requires thoughtful progression, attention to intensity, and integration of recovery strategies.

With the **360 Strategic Training** framework, endurance becomes a purposeful process where every mile serves a specific goal. By focusing on the quality of training—balancing intensity, managing stress, and incorporating recovery—you'll build a strong, resilient foundation for triathlon success.

Race Skills: Confidence for Race Day

Race day isn't just a test of fitness—it's where preparation meets execution. Race skills encompass the practical strategies and techniques needed to navigate the specific demands of your event. These skills help you stay calm under pressure, adapt to unexpected challenges, and maximize your performance.

The Importance of Race-Specific Practice

Preparation for race day begins long before the event. Practicing race-specific scenarios ensures you build not only competence but also confidence. The more you practice these skills, the more automatic they become, allowing you to focus on executing your plan and enjoying the experience.

Key Aspects of Race Skills

Race-specific skills vary depending on the event and conditions, but here are some of the most common and impactful areas to focus on:

- **Navigating Open Water:** Mastering sighting, swimming in high swells, and managing currents ensures you stay on course in challenging conditions. For ocean races, learning how to enter and exit waves effectively can save energy and time.

- **Cycling Proficiency:** Long stretches in the aero position, especially in headwinds, require not just physical strength but mental focus and practiced stability.

Knowing how to drink and eat in crosswinds or on technical descents ensures proper fueling while staying safe.

- **Hill Management:** Understanding when to stay seated or stand up during climbs helps you conserve energy and maintain power. Downhill techniques, such as staying aero while controlling speed, are equally important for technical courses.

- **Hot and Humid Conditions:** Racing in extreme weather demands careful pacing, hydration strategies, and heat management. Incorporating heat adaptation into your training helps your body perform in these conditions.

- **Transitions:** Quick, smooth transitions can shave minutes off your total time. Practicing the flow from swim to bike and bike to run ensures efficiency under pressure.

Note: These are just a few examples of race-specific skills. Depending on your race, there may be other factors to prepare for, such as altitude, cold water swims, or technical bike courses. A coach can help you identify and practice the unique skills required for your event, ensuring that no detail is overlooked.

Studying and Understanding the Race Course

Every race is unique, and familiarity with the course can make a significant difference. Key elements to research include:

- **Terrain:** Know the elevation profile, technical sections, and potential bottlenecks.

- **Weather Conditions:** Be prepared for factors like strong winds, heat, or sudden temperature changes.

- **Aid Stations:** Understand their locations and what's offered to plan your nutrition and hydration effectively.

- **Rules and Logistics:** Familiarize yourself with race regulations, cutoff times, and the layout of transition areas.

A coach is invaluable in this process, helping you identify blind spots and create a personalized plan that leaves nothing to chance. They can guide you through race simulations and provide feedback on your execution, ensuring you're ready for every scenario.

Building Confidence Through Practice

Confidence on race day comes from knowing you've prepared for every possibility. Regular practice of race skills not only sharpens your abilities but also reduces anxiety, allowing you to perform with clarity and focus. With the 360 Strategic Training approach, these skills are integrated into your training plan from the start—not as an afterthought. This ensures you're race-ready well before the big day.

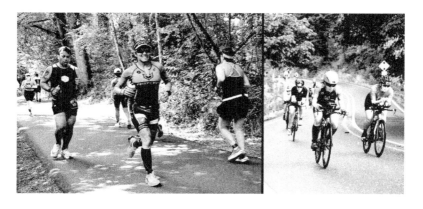

Why It Works

- Many athletes train solely for **distance**, which overlooks key elements like technique and speed that create sustainable performance.

- This approach targets **all aspects of athletic development**, ensuring not just completion but optimization of your race efforts.

- By addressing both the physical and tactical aspects of triathlon, it provides a comprehensive preparation plan.

How Smart Training Method and 360 Strategic Training Work Together

The **Feisty Fox Smart Training Method** provides the guiding principles, while **360 Strategic Training** focuses on the practical execution of each workout.

When combined, the Smart Training Method and 360 Strategic Training create a comprehensive, personalized approach to triathlon training. Here's how the synergy works:

- **Efficiency Over Volume:**

  - The Smart Training Method emphasizes quality over quantity, ensuring your efforts are targeted and intentional.

  - 360 Strategic Training takes this further by focusing on the most effective techniques, paces, and skills for each session, minimizing wasted energy and maximizing gains.

- **Injury Prevention:**

  - The Smart Training Method prioritizes injury prevention through body maintenance, gradual progression, and recovery practices.

  - 360 Strategic Training reinforces this by fine-tuning your form and technique, reducing strain on your body and addressing weaknesses before they lead to setbacks.

- **Balanced Development:**

  - The Smart Training Method addresses all aspects of your life—training, work, family, and recovery—ensuring sustainable progress.

  - 360 Strategic Training balances physical and technical development, so you're not just training to complete distances but to excel in all three disciplines.

- **Confidence Through Preparation:**

  - The Smart Training Method instills confidence by creating a solid foundation through tailored workouts and structured guidance.

- 360 Strategic Training builds on this by providing race-specific skills and simulations, so you feel prepared for any challenge on race day.

- **Sustainability and Longevity:**

  - The Smart Training Method helps athletes achieve their goals without compromising their health or life balance, fostering a long-term love for the sport.

  - 360 Strategic Training ensures ongoing improvement by continually adapting to your needs and goals, preventing plateaus and keeping your journey exciting.

  - Training smarter means prioritizing your body's needs so you can perform at your best—not just for one race but for years to come. This approach isn't about training harder; it's about training smarter through structured techniques, body maintenance, and recovery strategies.

Later in this book, we'll explore these elements in greater detail, helping you build a foundation for long-term success and a love for triathlon and endurance sports that lasts a lifetime.

FREE GIFT: 360 Strategic Training Overview Worksheet

Training for a triathlon and endurance sports can feel overwhelming, but it doesn't have to be! I'm giving you the **360 Strategic Training Overview Worksheet** to help you focus on what really matters:

- Technique

- Speed and pacing

- Endurance

- Race-specific skills

This worksheet will guide you to train smarter, avoid burnout, and get race-day ready with confidence.

How to Get It:

Scan the QR code below or visit <u>bit.ly/free-gifts-unstoppable</u> to download your free copy.

With this tool, you'll be training like a pro in no time. Let's make your next finish line your strongest yet!

SCAN ME

Chapter 2 Summary: Stay Injury Free - Training Smarter, Not Harder

Key Insight: Injury-free training isn't about pushing harder—it's about training smarter. By focusing on balance, structured plans, proper technique, and recovery, athletes can achieve their goals while fostering longevity in the sport. The Feisty Fox Smart Training Method and 360 Strategic Training emphasize a comprehensive approach that integrates physical preparation, mental fitness, nutrition, and race-day strategy.

Core Strategies

- **Training** - Structured, personalized workouts

- **Nutrition** - Personalized fueling to support recovery and energy.

- **Body Maintenance** - Strengthening weak areas, addressing imbalances and promoting quickly.

- **Mental fitness** - Building resilience and discipline

- **Race Strategies** - Preparing for race-day challenges with detailed plans

- **360 Strategic Training**

  - Integrates technique, speed, endurance, and race specific skills to train efficiently and confidently.

  - Focuses on training efficiency rather than sheer volume.

- **Personalized Plans:** Use tailored strategies that adapt to your daily realities, stress levels, and feedback.

- **Holistic Monitoring:** Track both physical and mental metrics—fatigue, soreness, and mental clarity—to refine your approach.

Actionable Steps

- **Prioritize Technique:**

    a. Focus on efficient swim strokes, proper running form, and cycling cadence.

    b. Seek feedback through video analysis or coaching to correct inefficiencies.

- **Implement Body Maintenance:**

    a. Incorporate regular soft tissue care maintenance, mobility, strength and functional exercises

- **Schedule active recovery days and adequate sleep.**

- **Adopt a Personalized Training Plan:**

    a. Use tailored plans that adjust to your stress, fatigue, and daily realities.

- **Monitor Progress:**

    a. Track physical and mental feedback in a journal or app.

    b. Use data like pace, power, and perceived effort to refine your approach.

- **Communicate with your Coach:**

    a. Share specific details about discomfort or fatigue to enable real-time plan adjustments.

Reflection Questions

1. What steps am I taking to prevent injuries and address weak areas in my body?

2. Do I understand the purpose behind each workout, and how does it align with my goals?

3. How well do I balance training intensity with recovery?

4. What signs of fatigue or discomfort have I noticed recently, and how can I address them?

5. Am I incorporating body maintenance and mental fitness into my routine?

Chapter 3

Key Strategies for Training Smarter

Excellence is never an accident. It is always the result of high intention, sincere effort, and intelligent execution.

– Aristotle

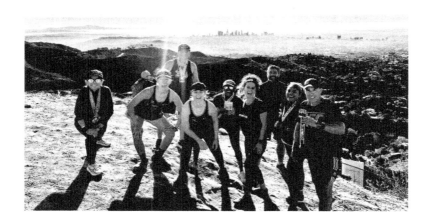

I used to think that training success was all about logging more hours and pushing harder, but I quickly learned the hard way that it wasn't sustainable.

During my preparation for one of my early triathlons, I was cramming long workouts into an already packed schedule. I thought the more I trained, the better I'd get. But instead of seeing improvement, I felt burnt out and frustrated because I wasn't hitting my goals. That's when I made a critical shift. I started focusing on what really mattered: quality over quantity. I traded endless junk miles for purposeful, high-impact sessions. Each workout had a specific goal—whether it was improving technique, building endurance, or sharpening race skills. That change didn't just transform my training; it transformed my confidence.

Later in my career, this lesson was tested in ways I never expected. One of the things I wish I had understood earlier is that getting faster and stronger isn't about simply going longer or logging more hours. This truth hit home when I faced the challenge of training for an unplanned Guinness World Record attempt. I went on to complete 5 Ironman races in 5 consecutive days, finishing with the fastest time.

People often ask me, 'How did you do it?' The answer lies in everything I had learned about smart training:

- ***Targeted workouts** that focused on building strength and speed without overtraining.*

- ***Efficient recovery routines** to keep my body fresh for back-to-back races.*

- ***Laser focus on technique and pacing**, ensuring every swim, bike, and run had a purpose.*

Training smarter, not longer, allowed me to achieve what once felt impossible. It wasn't about sacrificing every hour of my life—it was about making every hour of training count. When you train with intention and execute intelligently, you unlock a level of performance you never thought possible. Excellence is never an accident—it's the result of a smart, focused plan and the determination to stick to it.

– Coach Shangrila

To train smarter—not harder—we emphasize the following practical strategies, grounded in the principles of **Smart Training** and **360 Strategic Training.**

1. Technique Refinement: Build Efficiency

Small adjustments in how you swim, bike, or run can make a significant difference. Good technique reduces strain, improves efficiency, and lowers injury risk:

- **Swimming**: Perfect your stroke mechanics, body position, and breathing rhythm to reduce drag and conserve energy.

- **Cycling**: Dial in your bike fit, pedal stroke, and cadence to improve power output and avoid overuse injuries.

- **Running**: Optimize your stride length, foot strike, and posture to minimize impact stress and improve efficiency.

2. Body Awareness: Listen to Your Body

Developing body awareness is a critical skill for triathletes aiming to train effectively, prevent injuries, and achieve long-term success. Your body constantly sends signals about its condition during and after workouts—it's up to you to interpret and act on them wisely.

Understand Training Fatigue vs. Pain

One of the most important distinctions to make is between normal training fatigue and pain that could signal injury:

- **Training Fatigue**: Mild soreness, muscle tightness, or general tiredness after a workout is normal. It's part of the recovery process as your body adapts to training.

- **Pain or Injury Signals**: Sharp, persistent, or localized pain, as well as unusual discomfort that doesn't subside with rest, may indicate an injury or overuse issue. Ignoring these warning signs can lead to long-term setbacks.

Identify Signs of Overtraining

Overtraining doesn't happen overnight—it's a gradual build-up of stress that exceeds your body's ability to recover. Look out for common signs such as:

- Persistent fatigue that doesn't improve with rest.

- Poor performance, even during routine workouts.

- Increased irritability, mood swings, or lack of motivation.

- Disturbed sleep or difficulty concentrating.

Addressing these symptoms early can prevent burnout and allow you to maintain consistent, productive training.

Communicate Openly with Your Coach

Coaches rely on feedback from their athletes to adjust training plans effectively. If you experience discomfort, fatigue, or changes in your performance:

- **Don't hesitate to speak up.** Open communication with your coach helps identify potential problems early and ensures your training plan aligns with your current state.

- **Share specific details.** Explain when discomfort occurs, how severe it is, and any patterns you've noticed. This information helps your coach make informed decisions to prevent setbacks.

Body Awareness: Listen to Your Body

Developing self-awareness is critical for any athlete, whether working with a coach or managing training independently. A coach can help you interpret and act on your body's signals more effectively, but if you're training solo, self-monitoring becomes even more essential.

- **Keep Detailed Records:** Tracking your workouts and recovery patterns can help you identify trends and adjust your training.

- **Seek Feedback:** Even without a dedicated coach, consulting experts or peers can help prevent blind spots in your training.

- **Educate Yourself:** Learn the basics of technique, recovery, and progression to avoid common mistakes and make informed decisions.

While self-training can help you progress, it often involves trial and error. A coach eliminates much of this guesswork, accelerating your growth and ensuring your training aligns with your goals. Even as an experienced coach, I still seek guidance from other professionals to uncover blind spots and achieve my own goals efficiently.

3. Recovery: Make Time for Growth

Why Recovery Is More Than Soreness

Soreness is just one indicator of stress on your body, specifically within the muscular system. However, triathlon training and racing demand more than muscular output. High-intensity workouts, long training sessions, or endurance races also tax your **cardiovascular system**, **nervous system**, and **immune system**, among others.

Neglecting to evaluate recovery holistically can result in:

- Lingering fatigue that compromises future training sessions.

- Subtle, accumulating stress that leads to overtraining or injury.

- Suppressed immune function, leaving you vulnerable to illness.

- Poor adaptations, limiting your performance gains.

What Complete Recovery Looks Like

A proper recovery plan ensures that **every system** in your body has had time to heal, recharge, and adapt:

Physical Recovery

- **Muscular Recovery:** Microtears in your muscles from training heal during recovery, making you stronger. However, this process requires not just rest but also proper nutrition to rebuild tissues.

- **Cardiovascular Recovery:** Your heart and blood vessels work overtime during endurance sessions. Overtraining without rest can lead to decreased efficiency and even prolonged heart strain.

- **Nervous System Recovery:** Hard sessions stimulate your central nervous system, which governs motor skills, coordination, and response time. Without adequate rest, this system becomes fatigued, affecting both performance and mental sharpness.

Hormonal & Immune Recovery

- **Hormonal Recovery:** Hormones like cortisol and adrenaline spike during training and racing. Without recovery, chronic elevation of these stress hormones can lead to burnout or fatigue.

- **Immune System Recovery:** Long sessions, especially in hot or cold conditions, can temporarily weaken your immune defenses, making you more susceptible to illness.

Recovery Tools and Strategies

- **Rest Days:** Schedule at least one full rest day per week to allow your body to heal and adapt. These breaks aren't lazy—they're an essential part of becoming stronger and faster.

- **Active Recovery:** Include low-intensity activities like yoga, walking, or light swimming to promote blood flow and speed up the clearance of metabolic waste.

- **Sleep:** Aim for 7-9 hours of high-quality sleep per night. Sleep is when your body performs critical repair processes, such as muscle rebuilding, memory consolidation, and immune system strengthening.

Nutritional Recovery

- **Nutrition:** Focus on replenishing glycogen stores and repairing muscles with adequate carbohydrates, proteins, and micronutrients. Aim for anti-inflammatory foods like leafy greens, berries, salmon, walnuts, and turmeric to reduce inflammation and promote faster recovery. Hydration is equally crucial for cellular repair and function.

Monitoring and Listening to Your Body

- **Monitor Biomarkers:** Pay attention to more subtle recovery markers such as resting heart rate, variability in heart rate (HRV), mood, and energy levels. A well-recovered body will exhibit stable energy, consistent heart rate, and positive mood.

- **Listen to Your Body Beyond Soreness:** Fatigue, poor performance, and lack of enthusiasm for training can all indicate insufficient recovery, even if you're not sore.

Recovery Is Training

Recovery isn't a passive part of your plan—it's an active component of your success. Failing to recover fully, especially after long or intense sessions, undermines the adaptations that make you stronger, faster, and more resilient. Remember, you don't get stronger during training—you get stronger during recovery. By prioritizing recovery for all your systems and fueling with anti-inflammatory foods, you'll unlock your body's full potential and set the stage for consistent progress.

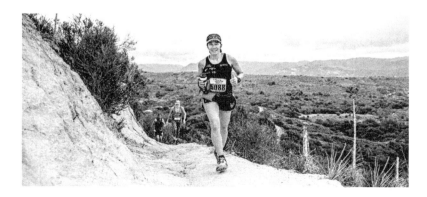

4. Progress Gradually: Avoid Overtraining

The **10% Rule** is a commonly used guideline to prevent overtraining. It suggests increasing your weekly training volume—measured by time or distance—by no more than 10% per week.

A study published in the *Journal of Sports Science and Medicine* (van Mechelen et al., 1992) supports the 10% rule, suggesting gradual increases in training volume to minimize the risk of overuse injuries. Incremental progress allows the body to adapt without overloading joints, tendons, or muscles.

For example:

- **By Time:** If you train for 6 hours in one week, aim for 6 hours and 36 minutes the next week.

- **By Distance:** If your weekly run mileage is 20 miles, increase to 22 miles the following week.

While this is a helpful baseline, it's important to remember that it's just a guideline. Your unique circumstances—such as fitness level, recovery rate, and training intensity—play a significant role in determining how much you can safely progress.

Balancing Intensity and Volume

Increasing both intensity and volume at the same time can quickly overwhelm your body. To strike the right balance:

1. **Alternate Focus Areas:** If you're adding intensity, like interval sessions or hill repeats, keep volume stable that week. Conversely, when increasing volume, prioritize lower-intensity workouts (e.g., Zone 2).

2. **Use Intensity Strategically:** Incorporate harder sessions sparingly, ensuring your overall training load allows for adequate recovery.

3. **Monitor Training Load:** Use tools like Rate of Perceived Exertion (RPE) to assess how hard each session feels and track your overall workload. This subjective feedback helps you stay within your body's capacity and avoid pushing beyond safe limits.

Special Considerations for Unique Athletes

For athletes with additional challenges—such as injury-prone histories, ambitious goals like aiming to podium, USAT Nationals or world championship qualification, or training for multiple disciplines or races—progression needs to be even more calculated:

- **Injury-Prone or Recovering Athletes:** Pay close attention to discomfort or fatigue signals. Recovery and body maintenance routines become even more critical.

- **Combining Goals:** If training for multiple events (e.g., a marathon and a 70.3), rotate focus weeks to manage stress across disciplines.

- **Advanced Goals:** Athletes aiming for podium finishes or world championships require highly specific training blocks with strategic periodization, balancing race-specific intensity and recovery.

Balancing Complexity for High Achievers

Designing workouts for athletes who aim to achieve multiple ambitious goals within a short time frame requires a meticulous approach. I've worked with athletes who faced unique time constraints, injuries, and the pressure of pursuing overlapping milestones. These cases demand both creativity and precision in training plans.

Examples of High Achieving Athletes:

- **Hendrick**: A father of three with a full-time job, Hendrick faced two bulging discs causing sciatica during long runs and a torn rotator cuff tendon in his left shoulder. Despite limited time to train, he wanted to qualify for Boston in 3 months and complete his first full Ironman just 2 months later.

  - **Results**: Boston Marathon qualifier with a 3:21 time and a sub-15-hour Ironman finish in just 5 months.

- **Ngina**: A single mom in her 50s, Ngina tackled a 100-mile ultra run at Zion just 7 days after a PR performance at the 70.3 Oceanside. She not only excelled but won her age group in the ultra.

  - **Results**: 70.3 PR and AG win in her ultra within the same week.

- **Scott**: Scott achieved an Ironman 70.3 PR of 5:37:48 and completed the Boston Marathon just 10 days later, showcasing the results of calculated intensity and smart recovery strategies.

The Importance of Strategic Planning

These athletes' achievements weren't random—they were the result of tailored, complex training plans that accounted for their unique challenges and compressed timelines. High-achieving athletes often need:

- **Customized Periodization**: To ensure each phase builds on the last while allowing adequate recovery.

- **Targeted Recovery Strategies**: Intensive recovery practices, like foam rolling, yoga, and nutrition protocols, to manage accumulated fatigue.

- **Precision in Workouts**: Combining multiple goals in a single workout where appropriate, such as running off the bike or high-effort interval sessions.

- **Data-Driven Adjustments**: Using metrics like heart rate, power, pacing, and perceived effort to adapt plans in real time.

These examples illustrate how a well-designed approach enables even the busiest, most ambitious athletes to excel across seemingly incompatible goals.

Structured Training for Sustainable Progress

Effective training isn't just about working hard—it's about working smart. By balancing workload, intensity, and recovery, athletes can progress steadily while minimizing the risk of injury or burnout. The key principles of structured training include:

- **Foundational Development**: Begin with lower-intensity, consistent workouts to improve endurance and technique. This creates a solid fitness base for more challenging sessions later.

- **Gradual Progression**: Fitness gains require incremental increases in intensity and complexity. Incorporating speed sessions or intervals at the right time ensures progress without overloading your body.

- **Race-Specific Preparation**: Each race presents unique demands—whether it's navigating hills, mastering open-water swims, or achieving perfect pacing. Mimicking these challenges in training prepares you for race day success.

- **Planned Recovery**: Recovery isn't optional—it's critical for getting stronger. Strategic recovery periods allow your body to adapt, consolidate gains, and avoid burnout.

The Role of Expert Guidance

While these principles provide a foundation, experienced guidance ensures that your plan adapts to your evolving fitness, life demands, and external factors like stress and sleep.

- **Beyond the Numbers**: Metrics like heart rate, pace, and power are valuable, but they don't tell the whole story. External factors like work and family stress play a role in your capacity to train.

- **Preventing Mistakes**: It's easy to ignore early signs of fatigue or overtraining. An outside perspective can help you avoid setbacks and ensure you're progressing sustainably.

Even if you're self-coaching, keeping these principles in mind and staying adaptable to your needs can help you achieve steady, injury-free progress.

As one of my athletes, Erik, once shared, *"A good coach can change a game, a great coach can change a life."* This quote resonates deeply with the role coaching plays—not just in training smarter, but in transforming lives. Coaches don't just create training plans; they provide belief, accountability, and clarity that allow athletes to unlock their full potential. This is the reason so many athletes, even those with years of experience, seek out expert guidance—it's not just about the sport, it's about thriving in life.

Adjust Based on Feedback

Numbers are helpful, but they don't tell the full story. Factors like stress, sleep, travel, work and life demands can all affect your capacity to train. Pay attention to how you feel as training progresses:

- Persistent fatigue, irritability, or mood changes may signal the need for additional rest.

- Sharp or localized pain requires immediate action to avoid long-term issues.

- If in doubt, adjust your plan. Cutting back for a week is far better than risking injury.

A Holistic View of Progression

Progressing gradually doesn't just mean adding time or distance—it involves balancing volume, intensity, and recovery in a way that aligns with your goals, lifestyle, and personal limitations. This careful balance ensures that your body adapts effectively while minimizing the risk of injury or burnout.

For athletes juggling busy schedules, it may feel overwhelming to manage all these elements on your own. This is where a support system—whether it's a coach, training group, or knowledgeable peers—can be invaluable. They provide the accountability, expertise, and adjustments needed to keep you on track, even when life gets hectic.

Personally, I've found immense value in working with a coach for specific goals. It reduces frustration, uncovers blind spots, and accelerates the learning process by cutting out trial and error. With a coach's guidance, I can focus on my other commitments, knowing that my training is structured for success without me having to figure out every detail myself. It's an investment in not just your performance but your peace of mind.

The Takeaway

Gradual progression is about listening to your body, balancing workload, and respecting recovery. Whether you're a first-time triathlete or an experienced athlete chasing ambitious goals, the key is to adapt your training in a way that supports your growth while safeguarding your health. Remember, sustainable progress isn't a race—it's a thoughtful journey toward long-term success.

Chapter 3 Summary: Key Strategies for Training Smarter

Key Insight: Training smarter, not harder, involves refining your technique, listening to your body, and managing your recovery effectively. By focusing on incremental improvements and maintaining a balanced workload, athletes can achieve better results while avoiding burnout and injury.

Core Strategies

1. **Refine Swim, Bike and Run Technique**: Small adjustments to swim, bike, and run mechanics can significantly improve efficiency, reduce strain, and prevent injuries.

2. **Practice Body Awareness:** Learn to differentiate between normal fatigue and pain that signals potential injury. Recognizing these signals helps sustain long-term progress.

3. **Prioritize Recovery:** Recovery goes beyond rest; it includes muscular repair, cardiovascular regeneration, nervous system rebalancing, and hormonal recovery.

4. **Progress Gradually:** Adhere to sustainable training principles, such as the 10% Rule, to avoid overtraining and injury while maintaining consistency.

5. **Build a Support System**: Whether it's a coach, triathlon group, or online community, having support enhances accountability and reduces overwhelm.

Real-Life Inspiration: Athletes like Hendrick, Ngina, and Scott show how smart training helps you conquer challenges, juggle life's demands, and reach ambitious triathlon milestones.

Actionable Steps

- **Refine Swim, Bike, and Run Techniques**:

  a. Use video analysis or coaching to identify & correct inefficiencies.

  b. Incorporate drills targeting weak areas (e.g., high elbow catch for swimming, pedaling drills for cycling, stride length optimization for running).

- **Monitor Body Signals**:

  a. Keep a training log to track fatigue, soreness, and energy levels.

  b. Address sharp or persistent pain immediately with rest or professional input.

- **Plan Recovery Strategically**:

  a. Schedule one rest day per week and include active recovery sessions.

  b. Focus on nutrition for recovery—anti-inflammatory foods and proper hydration.

- **Use the 10% Rule**:

  a. Gradually increase training volume by no more than 10% per week.

  b. Alternate between high-intensity and low-intensity weeks to prevent overload.

- **Engage Your Support Network**:

  a. Share your progress and challenges with a coach or training partner.

  b. Join a triathlon group for advice, motivation, and camaraderie.

  c. Share your progress in our Free FB community so we can support and cheer you on! Here's the link: *https://www.facebook.com/groups/badass.triathletes/*

Reflection Questions

1. What specific aspects of my swimming, cycling, or running technique can I refine this week?

2. Am I recognizing the difference between normal training fatigue and signs of overtraining or injury?

3. How well am I incorporating recovery practices into my training routine?

4. Is my training plan progressing at a sustainable pace that aligns with my goals and energy levels?

5. Who can I lean on for accountability, guidance, or motivation in my training journey?

A Small Favor That Could Change Lives

Those who give freely, without expecting anything in return, create ripples of happiness and success in the lives of others—and their own. – Unknown

Hi, Athlete!

I've poured my heart into *Unstoppable: The Smart Training Method* with the hope that it helps you find balance, crush your goals, and live a healthier, more fulfilled life.

But now, I need your help. Not for me—but for someone like you. Someone who's just starting out, juggling life, work, and training, unsure of where to turn for guidance.

Every day, there are athletes struggling to find the right tools to train smarter, avoid burnout, and finally cross their finish line. These athletes could benefit from this book—*if they find it.*

This is where you come in.

<u>Would you take 60 seconds to help a fellow athlete?</u> Your review could be the reason they discover this resource.

Why Your Review Matters

Most people decide to pick up a book based on its reviews. Your feedback could inspire:

- **One more beginner athlete** to take their first step toward a healthier lifestyle.

- **One more parent** to balance their training without

sacrificing family or work.

- **One more triathlete** or **marathoner** to achieve a goal they once thought was impossible.

Your review can make a difference. Here's how to do it (it's super quick):

Head to the book's page on Amazon, click "Write a Review" and share your thoughts.

Share the Goodwill

If this book has helped you, share it with another athlete, a friend, or someone you know who could use a boost. You never know whose life you might change.

Thank you for being part of this journey. Your kindness, no matter how small, creates ripples that go far beyond what we can imagine.

SCAN ME
LEAVE AN
AMAZON
REVIEW

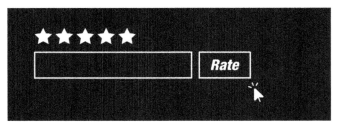

With gratitude,
Coach Shangrila
Your biggest fan and partner in crushing goals

P.S. Did you know that when you provide something of value to someone else, it makes you more valuable to them? If you think this book can help someone else, please send it their way. You might just be the reason they cross their first finish line—or achieve a goal they once thought was impossible.

Fun Fact: Helping others doesn't just feel good—it actually boosts your own happiness and success. So, thank you for making a difference! Now, back to your training.

Chapter 4

Body Maintenance & Injury Prevention

A good athlete knows their limits. A great athlete knows how to push them safely.

– Unknown

I used to not listen to my body. I thought some sniffles or a sore throat were no big deal, so I'd push through it.

One time, I showed up for a grueling King of the Mountain (KOM) century ride even though I wasn't feeling 100%. The next day, I raced a half marathon. My muscles felt fine, so I thought, 'Why not?'

Then, I decided to tackle some trail runs, reasoning that wrapping my neck with a warmer would make everything okay. I finished the workout, but I wasn't letting myself recover. I was making my body work harder than it should, ignoring the warning signs it was giving me. This wasn't just one isolated event—it was a pattern. Eventually, it caught up with me. I got so sick I couldn't do anything—I even had to call off work.

That was my wake-up call. I realized I wasn't just tired; I was overtraining. I had crossed the line from productive discomfort into destructive strain. Pushing harder wasn't making me stronger—it was making me weaker, draining my energy, and setting me back.

Since then, I've learned the difference between knowing your limits and pushing them safely. I became more proactive about my health, investigating my diet to focus on highly nutritious foods, prioritizing sleep, and managing stress. Most importantly, I started listening to my body. Now, when I feel the first signs of sniffles or fatigue, I think, 'Uh-oh, my body is telling me something.' My reaction isn't to push harder—it's to adjust: I hydrate more, eat better, get extra sleep, and lower my stress.

This experience taught me that great athletes don't ignore their bodies—they understand them. True performance comes from working with your body, not against it. When you listen to your body, you don't just recover—you stay consistent, avoid setbacks, and achieve long-term success. Because at the end of the day, it's not about reckless effort; it's about smart, intentional training.

– Coach Shangrila

In triathlon, consistent progress requires more than just completing workouts; it demands a strong, resilient body that can withstand the challenges of training and racing. However, the line between discomfort and injury is often blurred, leading athletes to either push too hard or avoid critical signals from their body.

This chapter delves into the tools and strategies for distinguishing discomfort from injury and explores the proactive steps you can take to maintain your body's health and strength. By prioritizing injury prevention and body maintenance, you're not just preparing for your next race—you're building a foundation for years of sustainable success.

Body Maintenance: Prevent Injuries and Stay Strong

What Is Body Maintenance?

Body maintenance is a proactive approach to keeping your body in optimal condition. It involves addressing weak areas, preventing injuries, and ensuring effective recovery. Think of it as essential upkeep—like brushing your teeth or changing your car's oil—to ensure long-term performance and health.

Understanding Discomfort vs. Injury

Knowing the difference between discomfort and pain is essential for injury-free training:

- **Discomfort**: Normal feelings of fatigue, tightness, or soreness during training adaptations.

- **Pain**: Sharp, sudden, or persistent sensations signaling something is wrong.

When you experience pain, follow these steps to prevent further harm:

1. Stop the activity immediately.

2. Gently stretch and massage the affected area to assess the severity.

3. Resume cautiously if the discomfort subsides. If the pain persists, consult a coach or medical professional for further guidance.

Key Components of Body Maintenance

Incorporating body maintenance into your routine prevents stiffness, improves strength, and enhances mobility and recovery. This includes:

- **Soft Tissue Care**: Use foam rollers or target trigger points to release muscle tension and improve recovery.

- **Strength and Stability**: Exercises that target glutes, core, and stabilizer muscles specific to your sport or activity.

- **Functional Movements**: Perform dynamic stretches and mobility drills to increase range of motion and prepare your body for training demands.

- **Active Recovery and Rest**: Allowing your body time to recharge and repair.

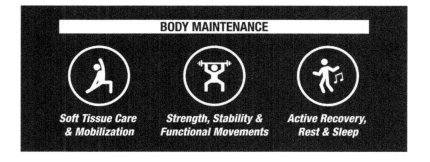

Why Stretching Alone Isn't Enough

Stretching is often seen as the cornerstone of recovery and injury prevention, but it addresses only one aspect of what your body truly needs. While stretching increases flexibility, it doesn't fully prepare your body for the demands of triathlon and endurance sports training or effectively prevent injuries. Incorporating mobilization, strength, and stability exercises provides a more comprehensive approach, targeting joint function, muscle control, and resilience.

1. The Limitations of Stretching

Static stretching focuses on muscle lengthening but fails to improve joint stability, neuromuscular control, or strength—all essential components for injury prevention. For example, a hamstring stretch might alleviate tightness temporarily, but it doesn't prepare the muscles and tendons for the repetitive stress of running or cycling.

2. Research Supports a Broader Approach

Scientific studies reinforce the need to go beyond stretching:

- The **Scandinavian Journal of Medicine & Science in Sports (2013)** found that static stretching alone did not significantly reduce injury rates in runners. Instead, injury prevention was more effective when dynamic mobilization and strength training were included to improve muscle control and joint stability.

- A study in the **British Journal of Sports Medicine (2018)** concluded that strength training can reduce injury risk by up to 50%. Building strength in muscles and tendons enhances resilience and improves shock absorption during high-impact activities.

3. Mobilization: The Missing Link

Mobilization drills are an often-overlooked yet critical component of an effective training and recovery plan. These dynamic movements actively improve **joint range of motion** while engaging stabilizing muscles, making them far more effective than static stretches alone. Unlike static stretching, which focuses solely on lengthening muscles, mobilization combines controlled movement and muscle activation to prepare the body for the demands of training.

Endurance athletes, particularly runners, cyclists, and swimmers, place repetitive stress on specific joints and muscle groups. Over time, this can lead to tightness, restricted mobility, and compensatory movement patterns, increasing the risk of overuse injuries. Mobilization drills help counteract these effects by ensuring that joints can move freely and efficiently through their full range of motion while activating the stabilizing muscles that support proper alignment.

A study published in the *Journal of Strength and Conditioning Research* (2019) found that incorporating dynamic mobilization drills before workouts led to **significant improvements in joint range of motion** and a notable reduction in injury risk for endurance athletes. The study demonstrated that mobilization not only enhanced flexibility but also primed muscles for activity, resulting in better muscle activation, reduced tightness, and improved overall performance. Athletes who included mobilization routines before training sessions reported fewer overuse injuries and improved movement efficiency.

How Mobilization Differs from Static Stretching:

- **Static Stretching** lengthens muscles but does not actively engage them. While it temporarily improves flexibility, it does not prepare joints or muscles for the dynamic movements of running, cycling, or swimming.

- **Mobilization** involves controlled, dynamic movements that mimic the motions of training. These drills not only improve flexibility but also activate key stabilizing muscles, increase blood flow, and enhance neuromuscular coordination.

Mobilization Practical Application:

Incorporating mobilization drills into your pre-workout routine takes only **5-10 minutes** but can significantly improve performance and injury prevention.

Ankle Mobilization Drill:

Purpose: Improves ankle dorsiflexion, enhances flexibility, and strengthens stabilizing muscles.

How to Perform:

1. Place one foot on a bench or step while keeping your heel planted.

2. Gently push your knee forward over your toes while keeping your foot flat.

3. Repeat for 10-15 controlled repetitions on each side.

Benefit: Prepares the ankle joint for the repetitive impact of running and cycling, reducing the risk of Achilles tendon or calf strain.

Hip Mobilization Drill:

Purpose: Improves hip flexibility, loosens tight hip flexors, and engages stabilizing glute muscles.

How to Perform:

1. Start in a deep lunge position with your back knee on the ground.

2. Rock your hips gently forward and backward, maintaining control.

3. Incorporate small circular motions to increase the range of motion.

4. Perform 10-15 repetitions on each leg.

Benefit: Prepares the hips for a full range of motion during running, cycling, or swimming, reducing tightness and improving stride efficiency.

Thoracic Spine Mobilization:

Purpose: Enhances upper back mobility, which is essential for swimming and maintaining good posture during cycling.

How to Perform:

1. Start in a kneeling position with your hands on the floor (child's pose).

2. Place one hand behind your head and rotate your torso, pointing your elbow upward.

3. Return to the starting position and repeat for 10-15 reps per side.

Benefit: Improves rotational movement in the upper body, enhancing swim stroke efficiency and reducing stiffness from long bike rides.

Why Mobilization Works:

Mobilization drills combine movement, flexibility, and muscle activation, which work together to:

- Reduce tightness in major joints.

- Prepare muscles for high-performance activity.

- Strengthen stabilizers to support efficient, injury-free movement.

By adding mobilization drills into your pre-workout routine, you not only reduce the risk of injury but also **unlock better performance** by ensuring your joints and muscles are primed for action.

Takeaway: Start every workout with a few key mobilization movements tailored to your sport. Whether it's the hips, ankles, or spine, these drills will keep you flexible, strong, and injury-resistant—ensuring you're ready to meet the demands of your training.

4. The Role of Strength and Stability

Strength and stability training address muscle imbalances and weak stabilizers—common contributors to injuries, particularly in endurance athletes. These imbalances often develop from repetitive movements such as running, cycling, and swimming, where certain muscles overcompensate for weaker ones. Over time, this leads to poor alignment, inefficient movement patterns, and a higher risk of overuse injuries.

Strengthening stabilizing muscles like the glutes, core, and ankle stabilizers is critical for maintaining proper posture, balance, and control during dynamic movements. Without sufficient stability, the body compensates in ways that place excess stress on joints, tendons, and muscles—ultimately leading to injury or plateaued performance.

According to a study published in the *Journal of Orthopaedic & Sports Physical Therapy* (2017), incorporating strength and stability exercises targeting the glutes, core, and stabilizers reduced lower limb injuries by **40%** in runners and cyclists. The study emphasized that addressing weak stabilizers early not only prevents injuries but also significantly enhances performance and resilience under physical stress. Strong stabilizers act as a foundation, enabling athletes to generate more power, maintain better form, and adapt to the physical demands of endurance sports.

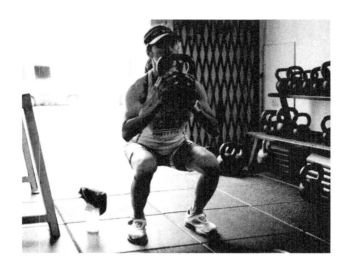

Strength & Stability Practical Application:

Target Key Stabilizers: Incorporate exercises that strengthen:

1. **Glutes**: Key for hip stability, power during running and cycling, and reducing knee injuries.
   Example: *Single-leg glute bridges* and *step-ups*.

2. **Core**: Enhances balance, posture, and energy transfer during movements.
   Example: *Planks*, *dead bugs*, and *bird-dogs*.

3. **Ankle Stabilizers**: Reduce injury risk by supporting proper foot strike and balance.
   Example: *Single-leg calf raises* and *ankle banded movements*.

Functional Movements: Perform compound exercises like lunges, squats, and single-leg deadlifts. These movements challenge multiple stabilizer muscles simultaneously, improving alignment and coordination.

Consistency and Progression: Incorporate 2-3 sessions of targeted strength and stability work per week. Start with bodyweight exercises, focusing on form and control, before progressing to resistance bands or weights.

By incorporating these elements, you create a body that is not just flexible but also strong, stable, and capable of adapting to the repetitive and dynamic demands of endurance training. A stable foundation reduces energy leaks during movement, enhances efficiency, and allows you to perform at your best while minimizing the risk of injury.

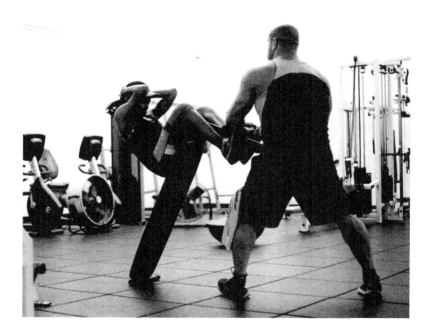

Chapter 4 Summary: Body Maintenance and Injury Prevention

Key Insight: Injury prevention requires proactive body maintenance, including strength training, mobility work, and addressing imbalances. Incorporating these practices into your routine supports long-term success in triathlon and minimizes disruptions caused by injury.

Core Strategies

1. **Understand Discomfort vs. Injury**: Recognize the difference between normal training fatigue and signs of injury.

2. **Strength and Stability Work**: Target weak areas like glutes, core, and stabilizers to improve overall performance and prevent overuse injuries.

3. **Body Maintenance Routine**: Incorporate foam rolling, dynamic stretches, and functional movements into weekly training.

4. **Active Recovery**: Use activities like light swimming, yoga, or walking to promote blood flow and accelerate recovery.

5. **Track Progress**: Keep a record of tightness, soreness, and energy levels to identify trends and areas that need attention.

Actionable Steps

- **Set Up a Body Maintenance Routine:**

  - Dedicate 15-20 minutes after workouts for foam rolling and stretches.

  - Use mobility tools to target tight areas (e.g., hips, IT bands, or shoulders).

- **Strength Training for Injury Prevention:**

  - Add two weekly sessions focused on glutes, core, and stabilizers.

  - Include bodyweight exercises like planks and glute bridges for beginners.

- **Monitor Tightness and Soreness:**

  - Use a journal to note recurring areas of discomfort.

  - Seek professional help (e.g., physical therapy) for unresolved issues.

- **Balance Rest and Recovery:**

  - Incorporate active recovery days to improve circulation.

  - Plan at least one complete rest day per week.

- **Educate Yourself**:

  - Watch videos or read resources about effective recovery and maintenance techniques.

  - Consult professionals for personalized advice.

Reflection Questions

1. How can I improve my current body maintenance routine?

2. Am I addressing areas of weakness or tightness before they escalate?

3. How do I differentiate between discomfort and pain?

4. Is my recovery plan sufficient to support my training volume?

5. What additional steps can I take to stay injury-free?

Chapter 5

Real-Life Transformations and Lessons

Every time you see greatness in someone else, it's your soul reminding you of your own potential.

– Unknown

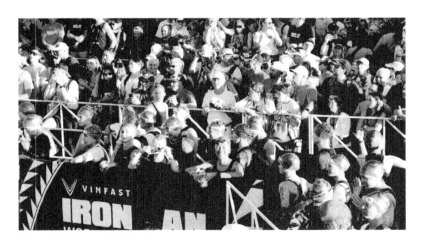

When I was new to triathlon, I remember how overwhelming it felt to juggle training, work, and life. There were days I doubted if I could handle it all. I'd think, 'Am I really cut out for this?' What helped me most wasn't just pushing harder in training—it was finding inspiration from others.

I started reading about Olympic champions, professional triathletes, and even everyday people who inspired me with their resilience. I listened to audiobooks and biographies of athletes and coaches, and I noticed something surprising: their challenges weren't so different from mine. Injuries, time constraints, self-doubt—they faced it all. Seeing that gave me a new perspective. I'd tell myself, 'If they can get through it, so can I.'

But it wasn't just about feeling inspired. I began studying their stories for patterns. How did they solve problems? How did they adapt when things didn't go as planned? I learned they didn't just work hard—they worked smart. They leaned on their support systems, made recovery a priority, and focused on small, consistent wins.

Their experiences became a guide for me. I started applying their lessons to my own training and life. Over time, I stopped seeing challenges as roadblocks and started seeing them as part of the process. I realized that the greatness I admired in others wasn't out of reach—it was something I could cultivate in myself.

Even now, when I face tough moments, I think back to those stories. They remind me that challenges don't define us—our response to them does. And it's a lesson I carry with me every day.

– Coach Shangrila

Claudia's Story: From Chronic Pain to Kona Finisher at 57

When Claudia began her journey, she faced an overwhelming list of physical challenges: **shoulder pain, back pain, plantar fasciitis, and chronic knee issues** that made back-to-back workouts feel impossible.

Her official diagnoses included **chronic patellofemoral maltracking, rotator cuff impingement, and tight hip flexors.** The idea of racing a full Ironman seemed completely out of reach.

Through the Feisty Fox Smart Training Method, Claudia turned these challenges into wins. We worked together to create a custom training plan tailored to her needs, focusing on addressing her physical limitations, strengthening weak points, and finding the root causes of her injuries. Consistent body maintenance, including soft tissue care, mobility drills, and targeted strength training, played a vital role in her transformation.

Today, Claudia is unstoppable. She made her Ironman comeback in New Zealand, finishing in 13 hours, conquered the Ultraman at 52, and recently crossed the finish line at the Ironman World Championship in Kona at age 57. But Claudia's journey doesn't end there—she's now one of our valued Feisty Fox coaches, sharing her story, teaching and inspiring others to overcome their own obstacles.

From being unsure if she could continue, Claudia has shown that persistence, smart training, and a strong mindset can lead to remarkable achievements.

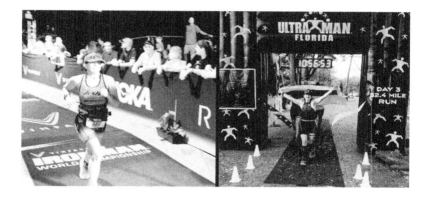

Bob's Story: Overcoming Age and Pain to Achieve New Heights

When Bob first reached out to Feisty Fox Coaching in his 60s, he was struggling with **persistent knee pain and felt like his age was catching up with him.** He worried that his best athletic years were behind him and couldn't see a way past the discomfort holding him back.

Through Feisty Fox Coaching, Bob embraced our Smart Training Method & 360 Strategic Training. We focused on refining his swimming, cycling, and running techniques, introduced structured workouts with targeted intervals, and prioritized body maintenance to address his knee pain and keep him injury-free.

Within just four months, Bob achieved incredible results:

- Comeback to racing 70.3 in Chattanooga: 5:27:17 (12th in his age group out of 107).

Fast forward, he continues to raise the bar each race, he achieved new milestones:

- A Half Marathon PR of 1:40:44 at age 63.

- Completion of 3 Ironman 70.3 races in a single season, including a PR of 5:20:34.

Bob's transformation shows that age is no barrier when you combine smart training, proper technique, and consistent body maintenance.

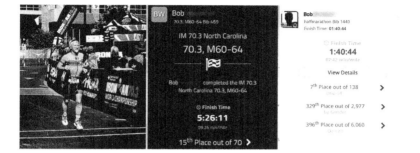

Scott's Story: From Injury-Prone to Setting PRs

Scott came to us with a long history of injuries—**plantar fasciitis, knee pain, bursitis, and hip issues.** These challenges, combined with a packed schedule of work and family commitments, made it difficult for him to train consistently or progress in his races.

The breakthrough came when Scott learned to identify the root causes of his pain. Rather than treating the symptoms, we worked on strengthening stabilizer muscles, improving body alignment, and balancing his workload to prevent overuse.

Over the course of just four months, Scott achieved the following milestones:

- Finished 5 races in 5 different states within 7 weeks.

- Achieved a 70.3 PR of 5:37:48 and finished the Boston Marathon in 3:46:52—within 10 days of each other.

- Qualified for the Boston Marathon for the 2x with a marathon PR of 3:06:15.

- In the same year, he also finished his first full Ironman with time of 11:30:16.

Building on this foundation, Scott later set even greater personal bests, including a new 70.3 PR of 5:15:20 and a half marathon PR of 1:31:20—all while staying healthy and confident in his training.

Scott's journey is one of resilience and smart adjustments. As he puts it,

"The places where I was hurting weren't the problem—they were the victims of imbalance. Fixing the root causes made all the difference."

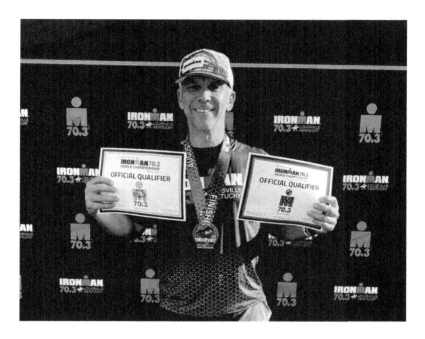

Jeremy's Story: From Spartan Races to Ironman & 8.2 miles Swim Success

Jeremy started with a bold dream: to complete an Ironman, but his journey was anything but straightforward. Coming from Spartan racing background, he **lacked experience in swimming and cycling.** In fact, he could **barely finish a single lap in the pool without gasping for air, and he hadn't ridden a bike since childhood.** Adding to these challenges were **frequent cramping issues and limited knowledge of nutrition.**

Despite these obstacles and a busy schedule balancing work, family, and his daughter's activities, Jeremy committed to the Feisty Fox Coaching program. He embraced structured training, focusing on consistency, proper technique, and smart nutrition. Over seven months, Jeremy achieved remarkable milestones:

- 3 months: Completed his first Olympic triathlon in 3:17:10.

- 5 months: Conquered his first 70.3—a hilly course—with a time of 6:26:54.

- 7 months: Finished his first full Ironman at Wisconsin in 15:12:45, with an impressive 2.4-mile swim time of 1:28:04.

The transformation didn't stop there. Within a year, Jeremy completed an 8.2-mile open-water swim around Mackinac Island—an accomplishment he couldn't have imagined when he first started. In the same eight-month period, he also completed his second 70.3 and second full Ironman.

Jeremy credits his success to staying consistent, giving 100% effort, and trusting the process. As he puts it:

"If I can do it, anybody can. It comes down to effort and consistency."

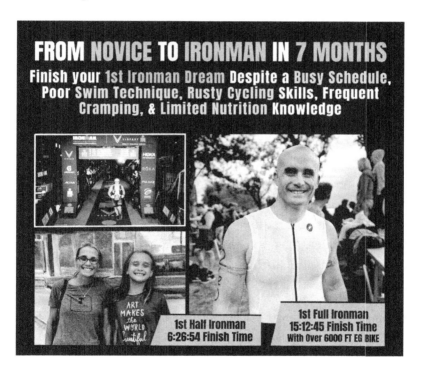

FROM NOVICE TO IRONMAN IN 7 MONTHS
Finish your 1st Ironman Dream Despite a Busy Schedule, Poor Swim Technique, Rusty Cycling Skills, Frequent Cramping, & Limited Nutrition Knowledge

1st Half Ironman
6:26:54 Finish Time

1st Full Ironman
15:12:45 Finish Time
With Over 6000 FT EG BIKE

Leo's Story: A Veteran's Journey to Overcome Injuries, 10 Surgeries, and Achieve Ironman Success

Leo, a proud veteran, faced extraordinary challenges on his journey to becoming a 2x Ironman finisher. With a medical history that included **back surgery, traumatic brain injury, PTSD, knee replacement, and shoulder surgery—alongside gout and chronic migraines**—Leo's story is one of perseverance, transformation, and a commitment to smarter training.

The Challenge: Rebuilding After Trauma

In 2018, Leo endured knee replacement and neck surgery just two weeks apart, leaving him unable to walk for months. It took him three years to regain his physical abilities, but his struggles didn't stop there. A back surgery in January 2022 brought new mental and physical hurdles. Leo knew he had to change his approach.

"I couldn't afford to train the wrong way again," Leo recalls. *"If I did it alone, I'd probably be back for another back surgery."*

A Smarter Approach to Training

Leo joined Feisty Fox Coaching determined to rebuild his body safely and efficiently. The first mindset shift came with understanding the importance of training smarter, not harder. "The biggest thing I learned was, don't train in pain," he explains. "Following the plan gave me confidence and kept me injury-free."

The program emphasized structured, progressive workouts tailored to his unique needs. Recovery was no longer an afterthought but a critical part of his strategy. This approach not only kept Leo healthy but also gave him the tools to rebuild his confidence.

Leo's dedication paid off; he finished his first full Ironman on the same year he had his back surgery. *"That last quarter mile was incredible,"* he recalls. *"All I could think about was the journey and how far I'd come."*

The following year, Leo achieved yet another milestone, completing Ironman Coeur d'Alene. His success wasn't just about the races; it was proof that the right mindset and system could turn obstacles into wins.

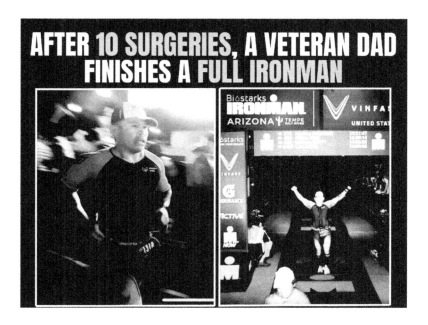

AFTER 10 SURGERIES, A VETERAN DAD FINISHES A FULL IRONMAN

Chapter 5 Summary: Real-Life Transformations and Lessons

Key Insight: Real-life athlete stories provide powerful inspiration and lessons, demonstrating how strategic training, proper mindset, and adaptability can overcome challenges and lead to remarkable achievements.

Core Strategies

1. **Learn from Others**: Study success stories to gain insights and motivation for your own journey.

2. **Identify Common Themes**: Look for patterns, like overcoming adversity, prioritizing consistency, or embracing flexibility in training.

3. **Adapt Lessons to Your Journey**: Apply what resonates with your challenges and goals.

4. **Celebrate Progress**: Acknowledge milestones, even small ones, as part of your larger success story.

5. **Stay Inspired**: Use these stories as fuel for tough training days or moments of doubt.

Real-Life Inspiration: Stories from athletes like Claudia, Bob, Leo and Scott show that smart training can help you overcome injuries, defy age, and achieve your triathlon goals.

Actionable Steps

- **Reflect on Transformation Stories**:

  - Note one lesson from each athlete that applies to your situation.

- **Celebrate Your Wins**:

  - List three recent accomplishments, no matter how small.

- **Create Your Success Vision**:

  - Write down how you want your training journey to inspire others.

- **Adapt Lessons**:

  - Identify one challenge you're currently facing and apply a lesson from the stories to overcome it.

- **Keep an Inspiration Log**:

  - Save quotes, stories, or milestones that motivate you.

Reflection Questions

1. What lesson from these stories resonates most with my current situation?

2. How have I already overcome challenges in my training?

3. What specific steps can I take to mirror the success of athletes I admire?

4. How can I celebrate my progress more effectively?

5. How can my journey inspire others?

What I Ask From You

This book was created to help you unlock your potential, and all I ask is:

1. **Read it with an open mind.** Whether you're new to endurance sports or a seasoned athlete, there's something here to help you reach the next level.

2. **Share your thoughts.** Let me know what resonated with you or what questions you have. Your feedback means the world to me!

3. **Pay it forward.** If you know someone who could benefit from this book, share it with them—it might just change their life.

Take Your Journey Even Further. Scan the QR Code Below to:

1. **Unlock exclusive Unstoppable book resources** to:

   a. Level up your swim, bike, run, and time management skills by applying the Smart Training Method and 360 Strategic Training tools from this book.

   b. Be inspired by real-life stories from athletes who overcame challenges, found solutions, and crushed their biggest goals.

   c. Dive deeper with step-by-step guidance through our coaching programs, tailored to help you implement these strategies into your life.

2. **Schedule a 15-minute Game Plan Call** to discuss your personal goals, identify the first steps to get you closer to achieving them and receive actionable advice tailored just for you.

Your best self - the strongest, healthiest and most empowered version of yourself is waiting. Let's get started.

RESERVE A
15 MIN
GAMEPLAN   GET MORE
RESOURCES

SCAN ME   SCAN ME

Chapter 6

Keeping Your Life Balanced - Redefining Success Without Sacrifices

"You don't have to sacrifice what matters to achieve your goals. Balance is not something you find; it's something you create."

– Unknown

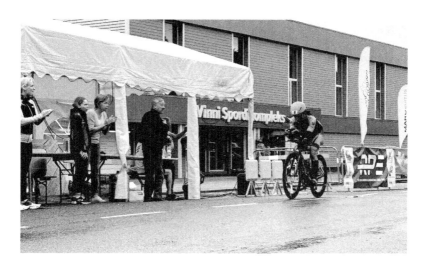

When I first started training for my first Ironman, I thought the only way to achieve my goals was to put everything else in my life on hold. I was working full-time, coaching athletes, and trying to manage my personal life, but it felt like I was constantly running out of time. I told myself, 'If I just push harder, I'll make it work.' But instead of feeling accomplished, I started feeling overwhelmed and disconnected from the people and things that mattered most to me.

I remember one specific weekend where it all came crashing down. I had back-to-back long workouts planned, but a family event popped up. I skipped the event to train, thinking it was the 'right' choice. But as I sat on my bike trainer later that day, I felt miserable. Sure, I was training, but I wasn't happy. I wasn't balanced.

That was a turning point for me. I realized I didn't have to sacrifice everything to achieve my goals—I just needed a smarter plan. I started aligning my priorities with my schedule: scheduling shorter, higher-quality sessions that fit around work and life, involving my family in active recovery days, and giving myself permission to take breaks when needed.

Now, balance isn't just something I strive for; it's something I create. I've learned that pursuing big goals is about integrating them into your life—not forcing your life to revolve around them. And the best part? When you make space for what matters, you enjoy the process so much more.

– Coach Shangrila

When you think of success in triathlon, the image of crossing the finish line, arms raised in triumph, might come to mind. But for many athletes—especially those juggling families, careers, and personal responsibilities—success goes far beyond race results.

True success is about finding harmony between training, work, and loved ones. It's about showing up as the best version of yourself—not just in the sport but in all areas of your life.

The Challenge:

Guilt and Self-Doubt

For many busy athletes, the challenge isn't just finding time to train—it's managing the guilt that comes with it. They worry that dedicating time to their goals takes away from their families or that prioritizing their well-being is selfish. But here's the **truth**: prioritizing yourself isn't selfish; it's essential. When done thoughtfully, triathlon training can enhance not only your life but also the lives of those around you.

This chapter is about **breaking the myths** surrounding guilt and self-care and discovering how triathlon can teach us valuable lessons about balance, resilience, and self-growth.

Life Balance Matters

The guilt is real. Many athletes feel torn between personal ambitions and their responsibilities at home. Kelly and Sarrah, two moms with busy schedules, once felt this way too. "How can I take care of myself when I have so many others to take care of?" they wondered.

Through trial, communication, and support, they discovered a life-changing truth: when they prioritized their health and happiness, they became better parents, partners, and role models. Their kids didn't just watch them train—they absorbed the lessons of discipline, perseverance, and joy.

Sarrah recalls her son saying, "Mom, you make me want to try harder in soccer." Kelly's children, inspired by her triathlon journey, even began signing up for kids' races.

The ripple effects were undeniable. Triathlon wasn't selfish. It became a way to teach their families the importance of self-care, pursuing goals, and showing resilience in the face of challenges.

Justin's Journey: Balancing Family, Business, and Triathlon Dreams

Justin, a husband and father of four young boys, juggled running a business with a 40-70 hour workweek while raising his family. After a five-year hiatus from training to prioritize his family and work, Justin decided to chase his ultimate goal: completing a full Ironman. However, he faced numerous challenges, including a history of knee injuries—a torn ACL and MCL with no meniscus in his left knee—and 15 extra pounds compared to his prime.

Working with Feisty Fox Coaching, Justin started with a clear goal: to finish his first Ironman injury-free. His coach emphasized intentional training that accommodated his busy schedule, from early morning workouts to efficient weekend training blocks. They incorporated body maintenance, strength, and stretching exercises to manage his knee discomfort and maintain his overall health.

Justin noted,

"The coaching pushed me hard enough to get it done, but was also understanding regarding my busy schedule with work and family balance. My coaches really knew how to cater the program to my ability and needs."

Through consistent effort and strategic planning, Justin finished his first Ironman in an impressive 12:51:14, crossing the finish line happy and injury-free. He went on to set personal bests in the 70.3 distance (5:58:04) and a half marathon (1:57:00). His wife, Kelly, and their sons played a crucial role, cheering him on during long workouts and even joining their local kids' triathlon events.

Justin's advice to others:

"You don't need all the gadgets. Just start. The right guidance, family support, and a clear plan will take you further than you thought possible."

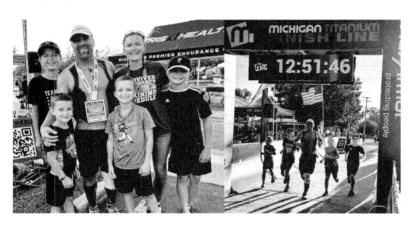

Zo's Journey: From Chronic Pain to Podium Finish & Pain-Free Milestones

Zo, a 58-year-old CrossFit trainer, water aerobics, and yoga instructor, faced a challenge that many athletes can relate to—persistent heel pain that wouldn't go away. For seven weeks, the pain in her heel radiated up to her knee, disrupting her training and daily life. Even during a hiking trip to Arizona, she dealt with cramping in her feet, pain in her Achilles, and shin discomfort. Despite her active lifestyle and mindfulness of her body, Zo couldn't find relief.

Like many athletes, Zo tried everything: sports massage, stretching, acupuncture, chiropractic care, physical therapy—you name it. But nothing seemed to work. "I didn't want a quick fix," she recalls. "I wanted to know what was wrong and fix it so it wouldn't happen again."

What she discovered was that isolated treatments were not enough. Stretching alone didn't address the deeper imbalances, and even strength training wasn't effective without proper structure. The key was integrating these elements into a proactive, personalized plan tailored to her specific needs as an athlete.

The Turning Point: A Holistic, Structured Approach

Zo decided to seek help from Feisty Fox Coaching because of its holistic approach.

"What I liked was how everything was connected—training, body maintenance, and accountability. That's what I needed to move forward," she said.

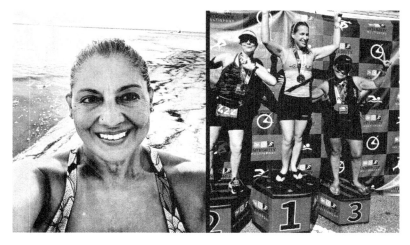

The coaching team evaluated not just her training routines but also her work as a yoga instructor and her daily activities. This holistic assessment revealed that her non-training activities, such as standing for long hours and improper footwear, were contributing to her pain. By addressing these external factors, alongside her training, she began to see improvement.

Key adjustments included:

- **Run Technique Refinement**: Poor form was aggravating her condition. Learning proper technique helped reduce strain on her heel and shin.

- **Structured Workouts**: Zo's training volume, intensity, and duration were restructured to balance stress and recovery, ensuring her body could heal and adapt.

- **Proactive Body Maintenance**: Regular soft tissue maintenance care, targeted strength exercises, dynamic stretches, and more were incorporated to strengthen weak areas and improve mobility.

- **Accountability and Communication**: Frequent check-ins ensured Zo stayed on track and adjusted her plan as needed.

The Result: Overcoming Pain and Achieving New Milestones

After eight weeks of structured, injury-free training, Zo not only overcame her heel pain but also finished third in her age group at the Fort de Soto Triathlon in Florida. "Although I didn't always understand the process, I trusted it," she said. "The accountability was great because it kept me focused, and I learned to listen to my body." Three months later, she achieved another milestone by running the most distance she'd ever completed—100 miles in a month—entirely pain-free!

Her story is a reminder that simply stretching or doing strength work isn't enough. Success lies in a comprehensive, proactive approach that incorporates proper technique, evaluates activities outside of training, and emphasizes high accountability. For athletes dealing with nagging injuries, Zo's journey proves that it's possible to come back stronger—and even achieve new milestones.

Solutions: Making It Work Without Sacrifice

1. Communicate with Your Family

Open communication is key. Kelly and Sarrah didn't just decide to train—they talked with their spouses, involved their kids, and made sure everyone understood why triathlon mattered to them. By sharing their goals and plans, they turned training into a family effort rather than a solo pursuit.

2. Integrate Training into Daily Life

Success doesn't have to come at the expense of family time. It's about training smarter and finding creative ways to integrate workouts into your routine.

Jeremy, for example, completed his early-morning runs, cycling sessions, or strength workouts while his family was still asleep. Sarrah found opportunities to train during her children's soccer practices, running laps near the field while they played.

The key is efficiency. By making the most of the time you have, you can maintain progress without missing important family moments.

Gwen: The Supermom of 5 Kids, Who Conquered Her Ironman Dream

Who dreams of completing a full Ironman while raising **five kids, ages 5 to 13, and working full-time?** Gwen did—and she made it happen with the unwavering support of her husband and a commitment to finding balance in her life.

Training for Ironman Arizona, Gwen averaged just 10 hours of training per week, with only two peak weeks reaching 12-14 hours. Her weekdays were carefully structured, with workouts lasting an hour each day (except Mondays, which were rest days). Weekends were reserved for longer sessions, but Gwen still made time for family gatherings, camping trips, birthdays, and holidays.

"I didn't feel that I missed being with my family," Gwen says. "I had to work out before they woke up, but I still picked them up, dropped them off, and stayed involved in their lives."

By communicating openly with her coach (me) and managing her time creatively, Gwen achieved her Ironman goal while staying injury-free and keeping her family life intact.

On race day, Gwen finished her first full Ironman strong, proving that with smart planning, dedication, and support, it's possible to achieve even the most ambitious dreams.Gwen's message to her coach sums it up beautifully:

"Thanks, Coach Shangrila. I share my medal with you. Thanks for helping me achieve this goal."

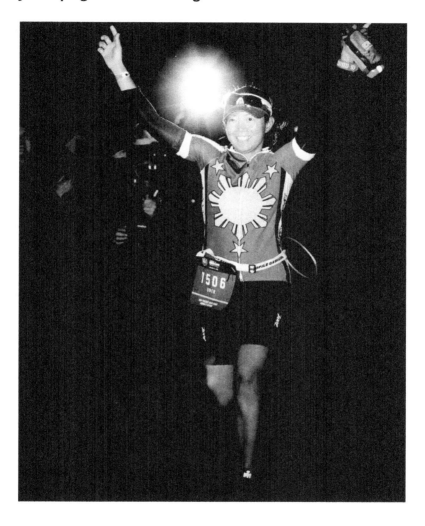

3. Set Boundaries and Schedule Intentionally

Boundaries are essential for maintaining balance. Sarrah made it a rule to dedicate Sundays to planning her children's activities for the week, ensuring their needs were met first. Jeremy and other athletes communicate their family events, work commitments, and time limitations with their coaches, allowing for tailored, flexible training plans that adapt to changing schedules.

By setting clear boundaries and prioritizing time management, athletes like Sarrah have been able to train effectively without disrupting their households. It's not about sacrificing one area of life for another; it's about designing a plan that works in harmony with your priorities.

Erik's Story: Qualifying for Kona While Balancing Life

For Erik, a father of four and a business owner, qualifying for the IRONMAN World Championship in Kona was more than just a physical accomplishment—it was a journey of mental growth, self-discovery, and mastering the art of balancing an ambitious goal with the demands of daily life. His story highlights the transformative power of preparation, resilience, and community in achieving big dreams.

Top Lessons From Erik's Journey

1. Mental Strength is Key *"The mental health aspects are just as important as the physical health,"* Erik explains. *"There are going to be times when you want to quit, but you have to strengthen your mind and make the choice that this is something you want to do."*

Erik learned that building mental resilience was essential to overcoming challenges and staying focused, even when self-doubt crept in.

2. Trust the Process and Your Coach Erik emphasizes the importance of coaching: *"There's a lot of conflicting advice out there, and without a coach, it's easy to get confused. Having someone who knows you and can push you beyond what you think you're capable of is invaluable."*

He also stresses the significance of trust, communication, and camaraderie with your coach. *"You need a coach who knows when to push and when to pull, and who helps you unlock potential you didn't know you had."*

3. Community Matters Through Feisty Fox Coaching, Erik found a supportive network of like-minded athletes who motivated him and shared in his triumphs and struggles. *"I've made incredible friends through this program—even people I've never met in person. The camaraderie and mutual encouragement are huge."*

4. Life Balance is Non-Negotiable Balancing training with life's demands was one of Erik's biggest takeaways. He learned to prioritize, communicate effectively with loved ones, and accept that his dream wasn't shared by everyone around him. *"You can't get angry when others don't share your dream. It's your goal, and you have to figure out how to make it work for you."*

Overcoming Challenges: Building Resilience

Erik didn't shy away from the hard days. He embraced the reality that progress doesn't always feel good. *"A third of the time, you'll feel great; a third of the time, so-so; and a third of the time, downright crappy. That's when the real growth happens."*

He also developed tools to overcome negative self-talk and focus on personal improvement rather than comparison. *"Be careful what you say to yourself. Self-talk can spiral quickly if you're not mindful. And if you're going to compare yourself to others, use it as inspiration—not discouragement."*

Staying Grounded: Reflection and Growth

After achieving his goal of qualifying for Kona, Erik took time to reassess.

"It's natural to want to keep grinding forward, but it's important to pause, reflect, and figure out where you want to go next. Your dream should scare you a little—if it doesn't, it's not big enough."

Erik's Advice for Balancing Life and Ambitious Goals

- **Lean on Support**: *"You'll need help along the way. Don't be afraid to ask for it."*

- **Prepare for Fatigue**: *"Growth happens in the fatigue. Recovery is where you gain strength."*

- **Embrace Challenges**: *"Your mindset matters. Growth lies in overcoming discomfort."*

- **Celebrate Wins**: *"Good luck finds those who are prepared, so always do your best and enjoy the journey."*

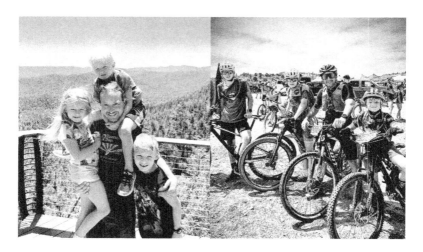

Reggie's Story: Balancing Family, Business, and Ironman Success

For Reggie, a father of three and busy business owner, the thought of completing a full Ironman seemed impossible. Juggling work, family, and training felt overwhelming. *"The thought of even finishing a full Ironman seemed like a huge mountain to climb,"* he admits. But by focusing on key strategies, Reggie transformed challenges into opportunities.

Breaking It Down: Overcoming the Daunting Challenge

Reggie faced the same doubts many athletes experience: juggling work, family, and training seemed impossible. His busy schedule included frequent travel, leaving little room for outdoor workouts. However, instead of succumbing to these obstacles, Reggie shifted his perspective.

"It's like anything in life—if you take it one step at a time and set micro-goals, you can break down even the biggest challenges," he shares.

By compartmentalizing his responsibilities and focusing on one goal at a time, Reggie stayed consistent.

He embraced indoor training, using tools like Zwift and treadmill sessions to maximize his time and efficiency. *"It's about putting in the work, whether it's indoors or outdoors. Consistent effort adds up,"* Reggie emphasizes.

The Ups and Downs: Growth in Nonlinear Progress

Reggie quickly learned that progress is rarely a straight line. *"It hasn't been linear,"* he admits. *"There are ups and downs, but as long as you're always making constant improvements, you can't go wrong."*

Small, consistent improvements—like shaving seconds off his swim time—gave him the motivation to keep pushing.

"Focusing on getting 1% better every day made a huge difference. Even if it doesn't feel like much at the moment, over time, those improvements are massive."

With coaching and data-driven feedback, Reggie refined his training approach. *"It's not just about working harder; it's about working smarter—knowing when to push and when to rest."*

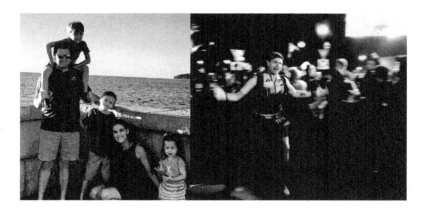

Balancing Family and Training

As a father, Reggie grappled with the emotional toll of spending time away from his children during long training sessions. *"When you're dedicating large blocks of time to training, it's easy to feel guilty as a parent,"* he says.

Reggie found a way to bridge the gap by involving his family in his journey. *"Getting my kids involved in the training process allowed me to stay connected with them and reduced the guilt. It also made them a part of the journey."*

His family began attending races, cheering him on, and celebrating his victories. *"When I cross the finish line, it's not just my victory—it's our tribe's victory. Everyone had a hand in it."*

Community: The Secret to Staying Motivated

Joining the Feisty Fox Coaching community kept Reggie motivated. *"Surrounding yourself with like-minded people who are better than you is crucial. They push you to improve and keep you accountable."* The camaraderie and shared goals provided the extra push he needed during challenging times.

Key Takeaways for Busy Athletes

Reggie's journey offers inspiration and practical advice for athletes balancing life's demands:

- **Set Clear Goals**: "Break big challenges into small steps. Micro-goals lead to big wins."

- **Work Smarter**: Use tools like indoor training and focus on quality over quantity.

- **Involve Your Family**: Including loved ones makes the journey more fulfilling.

- **Surround Yourself with Support**: A strong community or coach can elevate your performance.

Inspiring Others Through His Journey

Reggie's story proves that even the busiest athletes can achieve incredible results with the right mindset, support system, and willingness to adapt.

"The great thing about Ironman is that it's not supposed to be easy," he says. "But if you commit to it, there's no stopping you."

His journey reminds us that success doesn't require perfect conditions or a straight path—it's about determination, resourcefulness, and surrounding yourself with people who believe in your potential.

Inspiration: Redefining What Success Means

The traditional idea of success—winning races or hitting personal records—is only part of the story. For athletes like Kelly, Sarrah, Erik, Jeremy and Reggie, success is about becoming better versions of themselves. It's about **balancing** ambition with life's responsibilities and proving that you don't have to choose between personal goals and family.

As Sarrah once said,

"Triathlon isn't just about crossing the finish line. It's about the example I set for my kids—that it's okay to chase your dreams, even when life is busy."

So, if you've been hesitating to pursue your goals because you feel it's selfish or impossible, remember this: Triathlon isn't just about finishing races; it's about showing up as **your best self** for those you love. By investing in yourself, you inspire those around you to do the same. And that's a legacy worth creating.

The Takeaway: Success Without Sacrifice

Success in triathlon doesn't mean neglecting your family or overcommitting yourself. It's about creating a **sustainable** balance between training and life. When you focus on smart strategies—like open communication, efficient scheduling, and intentional boundaries—you can achieve your goals without sacrifice.

Triathlon has the power to **enrich** your life and **inspire** those around you. By redefining success, you're not just crossing finish lines—you're showing your family, friends, and community what's possible when you prioritize health, happiness, and balance.

That's a legacy worth creating.

Chapter 6 Summary: *Keeping Your Life Balanced - Redefining Success Without Sacrifices*

Key Insight: Success in triathlon isn't just about crossing the finish line—it's about balancing your personal goals with your responsibilities to family, work, and yourself. When done thoughtfully, pursuing triathlon can enrich all areas of your life and inspire those around you.

Core Strategies:

1. **Redefine Success**: Shift the focus from race results to the impact your journey has on your well-being and relationships.

2. **Communicate Openly**: Involve your family and loved ones in your goals, creating a shared sense of purpose and understanding.

3. **Train Efficiently**: Use tools and methods, like early-morning sessions or combining workouts, to maintain progress without disrupting family life.

4. **Set Boundaries**: Prioritize time management and clearly communicate your needs to avoid conflict or guilt.

5. **Involve Your Family**: Transform training into a family-inclusive activity that sets a positive example and strengthens your bond.

Real-Life Inspiration: Stories of athletes like Zo, Gwen, Erik, Sarrah, and Reggie highlight how effective communication, efficient training, and community support can turn challenges into opportunities for personal and family growth.

Actionable Steps

Take the following steps to redefine your triathlon success:

- **Define What Success Means to You**:

  - Write down what success looks like in triathlon and in your personal life.

  - Identify how these can complement each other rather than compete.

- **Communicate Your Goals**:

  - Share your aspirations with your family and explain why they matter to you.

  - Schedule a weekly family meeting to align plans and discuss support.

- **Make Training Family-Friendly**:

  - Find creative ways to involve your family, like running laps near your kids' soccer practices or riding on a trainer during family movie nights.

  - Celebrate milestones together, even small ones, as a shared achievement.

- **Establish Non-Negotiables:**

  - Set specific times for key life commitments (e.g., dinner with family or a weekly rest day) and stick to them.

- **Structure Your Week**:

  - Use a calendar to block out key training times that don't conflict with family or work commitments.

  - Prioritize rest and recovery to stay energized for all aspects of life.

- **Join a Supportive Community**:

  - Connect with other busy athletes through a coaching program, local triathlon groups, or online communities.

  - Join our Free FB community! Be the first to get FREE access to our new weekly live trainings about triathlon, nutrition, injury prevention, mental fitness and race strategy. Stay on track & get motivated by connecting with others. Join here: https://www.facebook.com/groups/badass.triathletes/

  - Use their encouragement and tips to stay motivated and balanced.

- **Reflect and Celebrate Small Wins:**

  - Each week, reflect on how well you balanced training and life, celebrating moments of harmony and identifying areas for improvement.

Reflection Questions

1. How do I currently define success, and is this definition aligned with my values?

2. What sacrifices am I making for training that could be avoided with better planning or flexibility?

3. How can I include my family or friends in my triathlon journey?

4. What strategies can I use to manage unexpected disruptions in my schedule?

5. What small wins can I celebrate this week to reinforce progress and balance?

Chapter 7
The Mindset of an Unstoppable Athlete

It always seems impossible until it's done.

– Nelson Mandela

Setting my second Guinness World Record—23 full Ironman-distance triathlons in 34 days—was one of the most grueling and rewarding experiences of my life. On my best day, I set a personal record of 13 hours and 10 minutes, with an unbelievable moving time of 11 hours 51 minutes. This included completing 55.2 miles swim, 2576 miles bike and 602.6 miles run while raising funds for 4 non-profit organizations and staying injury free. But getting to that point was anything but easy.

When the idea for the Beyond Myself Project first came to mind, it felt impossible. Completing 23 Ironmans was already an enormous challenge, but organizing a team of over 150 volunteers, coordinating logistics, and raising money for nonprofits made it feel almost unthinkable. I wasn't just pushing my physical limits; I was asking others to believe in a vision that was bigger than all of us.

The first few days were brutal. Freezing swims in the dark left me shivering, my knees ached on the bike, and I was so exhausted I started "sleep-cycling," moving my legs in pedaling motion while I dozed off. Every night, I'd collapse into the RV, barely able to walk, wondering, 'How can I possibly do another 140.6 miles tomorrow?'

But then, something extraordinary happened. My body adapted. What started as grueling, 15-hour races transformed into consistent sub-14-hour finishes. By the final weeks, I was stronger than I ever imagined. My comfortable run pace dropped from 11 minutes per mile to 9, and some days I even ran at an average of 8:30.

This project wasn't just about physical endurance—it was a testament to what's possible when you combine determination, teamwork, and belief in a greater purpose. If you want to dive deeper into how I achieved this record and the lessons I learned along the way, you can find the full story by scanning the QR code below.

It always seems impossible until it's done. And once it's done, you realize just how much you're capable of—and how many lives you can inspire by daring to dream big.

– Coach Shangrila

DAY	2.4 MI SWIM	112 MI BIKE	26.2 MI RUN	MOVING TIME	TOTAL TIME
1	1:46	6:44	4:55	13:25	15:59:23
2	1:51	6:29	4:47	13:07	15:52:30
3	1:53	6:41	4:35	13:09	15:39:24
4	1:46	8:12	5:37	15:35	16:28:09
5	2:06	7:39	5:42	15:27	16:53:00
6	1:38	9:08	5:47	16:33	17:48:00
7	1:38	8:07	5:50	15:35	17:13:55
8	1:34	7:39	5:45	14:58	16:27:31
9	1:36	7:12	5:48	14:36	18:02:01
10	1:35	6:53	5:57	14:25	17:00:41
11	1:30	6:36	5:17	13:23	14:27:38
12	1:29	6:47	4:41	12:57	14:28:54
13	1:30	6:40	5:05	13:15	14:30:00
14	1:31	6:16	4:58	12:45	14:49:12
15	1:28	6:50	4:38	12:56	13:54:12
16	1:32	5:58	4:25	11:55	13:46:05
17	1:29	6:18	4:05	11:52	13:49:01
18	1:31	6:19	4:17	12:07	13:32:13
19	1:29	6:39	4:13	12:21	13:19:35
20	1:31	6:10	4:29	12:10	13:10:24 PR
21	1:26	6:01	4:37	12:04	13:26:40
22	1:27	6:03	4:21	11:51	13:29:21
23	1:28	6:11	4:36	12:15	13:11:57

BEYOND MYSELF PROJECT

SCAN ME

The biggest challenges in triathlon aren't just physical—they're **mental**. Doubts creep in, whispering, "You're too old," "You're too busy," or "You don't have what it takes."

These voices can be louder than any hill climb or open-water swim. But here's the truth: Success in triathlon—and in life—starts with your mindset.

This chapter explores what it takes to overcome self-doubt, build resilience, and adopt the mindset of an unstoppable athlete. Because your mind is your greatest tool for achieving extraordinary goals.

Becoming World-Class: The Feisty Fox Vision

What does it mean to become *world-class*? It's not just about racing fast or hitting personal bests—it's about adopting a mindset and lifestyle that set you apart.

At Feisty Fox Coaching, we aim to create an army of world-class inspirational triathletes who crush their races while staying injury-free, maintaining life balance, and inspiring others.

Being world-class doesn't mean being perfect. It means striving to improve daily, showing resilience in the face of setbacks, and committing to your goals with consistency and purpose. It's about balancing ambition with gratitude, progress with patience, and hard work with self-care.

The Triathlete Mindset: Balancing Life, Training, and Self-Care

For busy triathletes juggling work, family, and personal goals, balance is the key to success. Your training should **complement** your life, not take it over. Achieving this balance requires a triathlete mindset grounded in these principles:

1. **Consistency Over Perfection**: You don't need to train every day or execute every workout perfectly. What matters is showing up regularly and focusing on small, meaningful progress. Success is built through consistent effort over time.

2. **Intentional Training**: Every workout should have a purpose. Are you working on technique, speed, endurance, or recovery? Aim for quality over quantity to avoid burnout and maximize your results.

3. **Body Awareness and Self-Compassion**: Listen to your body's signals. Pushing through pain is not a badge of honor—it's a recipe for injury. Adjust when needed, and respect the natural ebbs and flows of your energy and recovery.

4. **Adaptability**: Life happens. Meetings run late, kids get sick, or unexpected events arise. The key is flexibility—adapting your training plan rather than abandoning it. Stay coachable and open to adjustments when circumstances change.

5. **A Growth-Oriented Mindset**: View challenges as opportunities to grow. If a workout doesn't go as planned,

or if you miss a session, don't dwell on it. Instead, focus on what you can learn and how you can move forward.

6. **Patience and Positivity**: Progress in triathlon, like in life, takes time. Celebrate the small wins along the way and focus on what's within your control. Remember, the journey matters just as much as the destination.

From Zero Experience to Ironman in 9 Months: Gaye's Story

Gaye's journey from a complete beginner to an Ironman finisher in just 9 months proves that even the most ambitious goals are possible with the right plan and determination.

As a physical therapist, Gaye understood the human body but had **no endurance experience** and **doubted her ability to succeed** in triathlon. She started from scratch, **barely able to swim a single lap** and battling **thoracic spine pain** during freestyle. Coming from a hiking background, she had only recently completed her first full marathon with a time of about 5 hours. Her packed schedule, which included family commitments and travel to major marathons, made her question whether she could balance training while staying injury-free.

Despite these challenges, Gaye refused to let fear stop her. After completing Feisty Fox Coaching's 30-Day Swim Bootcamp, she gained the confidence to dream bigger. With a structured plan based on the Smart Training Method, she tackled technique, nutrition, pacing, endurance, race skills, and injury prevention - all while **training for 10 hours or less per week.**

She completed her first full Ironman **within 9 months of training,** all while balancing travel to the Berlin and London marathons.

- First sprint triathlon (April): She overcame her initial fears and doubts.

- First Olympic triathlon (June): Achieved a podium finish, placing 2nd in her age group.

- First 70.3 triathlon (September): Conquered ocean swimming with confidence.

- First full Ironman (October): Finished strong with a time of 13:30:08.

- Marathon PRs (April & October): Progressed from 4:56 to 4:16 across multiple races.

Gaye's ability to achieve so much in such a short period—while staying injury-free—demonstrates her dedication, adaptability, and willingness to trust the process. As a physical therapist, she also applied new techniques and strategies, enhancing her efficiency and results.

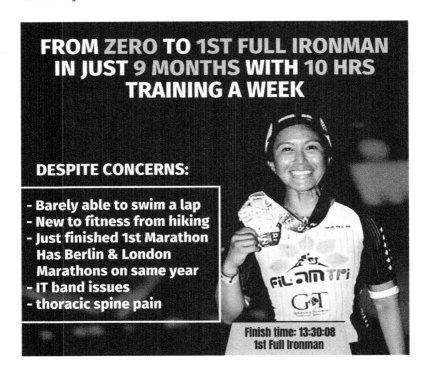

Reflecting on her journey, Gaye shares:

"This past year has been truly transformative, showing me that anything is possible when you're surrounded by a supportive community and expert guidance."

Her story proves that with a strong mindset, a personalized plan, and the right support, even the busiest athlete can achieve incredible results. Gaye didn't just conquer triathlon; she redefined what was possible for herself, inspiring others to do the same.

The Feisty Fox Manifesto: Defining the Unstoppable Athlete

A Feisty Fox is a **new breed of athlete**—smarter, healthier, stronger, and happier. Our athletes:

- Believe it's **never too late** to chase their dreams.

- **Fight against fears** and overcome limiting beliefs.

- Block negativity and **put in the work**, no matter what.

- Are **resourceful and result-driven**, finding ways to succeed without sacrificing health or relationships.

- Stay **committed** and execute their plans consistently.

- **Believe in themselves** so deeply, they keep trying, no matter what.

By embodying these traits, you can overcome any challenge and inspire others to do the same.

MANIFESTO

A Feisty Fox is a **NEW BREED OF ATHLETE.** *Smarter, healthier, stronger, happier and more determined.*

Feisty Foxes believe it's **NEVER TOO LATE** *to go after their dreams.*

Feisty Foxes **FIGHT AGAINST THE FEARS** *and limiting circumstances that hold most people back from trying.*

Feisty Foxes never make excuses. Instead they block negativity and **PUT IN THE WORK.** *They may fall short at times, but they will* **NEVER GIVE UP.**

Feisty Foxes are **RESULT–DRIVEN** *and* **RESOURCEFUL.** *They find ways to get results without sacrificing relationships, good health and longevity in training and racing.*

Feisty Foxes are **COMMITTED** *to keep raising the bar. They* **COMMUNICATE** *their values and execute* **CONSISTENTLY.**

Feisty Foxes **BELIEVE IN THEMSELVES** *so much, they will* **KEEP TRYING NO MATTER WHAT.**

I'M A FEISTY FOX

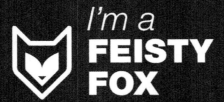

I'm a FEISTY FOX

I DEFINE my own limits

I CREATE my possibilities

I FACE my fears

I OVERCOME my weaknesses

I LIVE with passion

I INSPIRE OTHERS by my actions

I MOVE forward

I GIVE no excuses

---

*I CHOOSE not to be average,
because I am BEING MY BEST*

Champion's Mindset: Seiko's Journey to Qualifying for 70.3 & Full Ironman World Championships

When it comes to overcoming obstacles and embracing the mindset of an unstoppable athlete, few stories resonate more than Seiko's. A busy woman in her late 40s, Seiko juggled a physically demanding job, minimal swim access, and limited experience with endurance sports. Yet, she went on to qualify for both the Ironman and 70.3 World Championships—showcasing the power of mental strength, smart training, and determination.

Doubts and Challenges

Like many athletes, Seiko faced self-doubt at the beginning of her journey. With only one swim session per week and no prior experience in ocean swimming, she wondered if her goals were even achievable. Balancing work and recovery was also a significant challenge, as she noted, *"Some days at work were harder than race days. Recovery was crucial to avoid ruining both training and work performance."*

A Transformative Mindset

Seiko didn't let her doubts hold her back. She embraced the Smart Training Method, which focused on building not just physical strength but also mental resilience. By adopting a strategic approach, she turned challenges into opportunities:

- Visualization and Confidence: Watching demo videos and correcting her swim technique gave her the confidence to swim longer distances without pain.

"Learning proper technique reduced pressure on my shoulders and made me feel stronger with every stroke."

- Adaptability and Nutrition: Through training, she discovered personalized solutions for nutrition, including switching to rice and tea when sports drinks became unpalatable during long races.

- Patience and Recovery: Seiko viewed recovery as essential, not optional. *"If I'm not recovered, I can't train effectively, and that affects my overall progress."*

Outstanding Results

Seiko's journey highlights what's possible when mental and physical training align:

- Ironman 70.3 Gulf Coast: Finished in 5:42:36, earning a 22-minute PR and qualifying for the 70.3 World Championship.

- Ironman Chattanooga: Completed her first full Ironman w/ sub-13hrs finish time, placed 11th in her age group and earned a slot at the Ironman World Championship.

Her achievements came not from extraordinary circumstances but from consistent effort, belief, and the willingness to adapt. She says,

"This training program has made me healthier, happier, and more confident. I've learned that with the right support and mindset, even the busiest person can achieve incredible results."

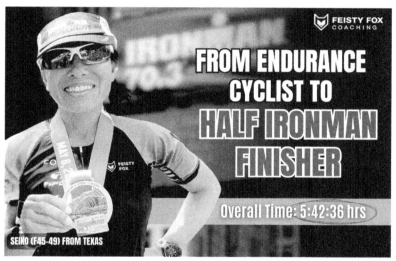

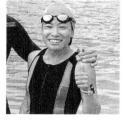
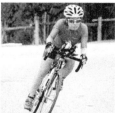
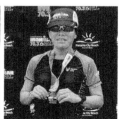

Lessons from Seiko's Story

Seiko's success teaches us three key lessons about mindset:

1. Recovery is Key: Treat recovery as seriously as your workouts to sustain progress and avoid burnout.

2. Embrace Visualization: Imagine yourself succeeding to build confidence and correct inefficiencies.

3. Stay Resilient: Focus on solutions rather than obstacles, and trust the process when the journey feels tough.

Amy's Story: Embracing New Challenges at 55 & Qualifying for 70.3 World Championship

Amy, a 55-year-old from Kentucky, is proof that mindset—not experience—defines your potential. Just a year ago, Amy was inspired watching her son finish a 70.3 race, but at the time, triathlon felt like a distant dream. She had no background in cycling, minimal understanding of the technical aspects of the sport, and doubts about whether she could handle the demands of training.

But Amy decided to go for it, signing up for her first 70.3 and trusting the Feisty Fox Coaching process. With a structured, personalized plan, she navigated the challenges step by step—building confidence, fitness, and mental resilience along the way.

Fast forward five months: Amy crossed the finish line at Ironman 70.3 Muncie with her family by her side, placing 9th in her age group and qualifying for the Ironman 70.3 World Championship in Spain.

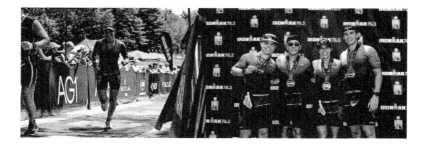

Lessons from Amy's Mindset Transformation

Amy didn't just train her body—she trained her mind, reshaping her outlook and approach to challenges. Here's what she learned along the way:

- **Trust the Process:** "It gets really, really hard at the end," Amy admits. "But I realized I was second-guessing myself unnecessarily. It turned out to be one of the most fun things I've ever done." Trusting her coach's plan and focusing on consistent effort helped her stay the course.

- **Celebrate the Journey:** For Amy, gratitude played a huge role. She thanked volunteers, police officers, and fellow athletes, finding joy in the experience. "Your attitude changes the whole outlook," she explains. "Mindset and physical performance go hand in hand."

- **Smarter, Not Harder:** Amy learned to avoid the "muscle-through" mentality.

"Triathlon isn't about grinding—it's about being efficient. Why work that hard unnecessarily when there's a better way to train?"

- **Community Matters:** The Feisty Fox tribe became a source of inspiration and motivation. "I loved seeing everyone's wins and knowing I wasn't alone in this journey. It reminded me to show up every day, even when it got tough."

A Milestone Worth Celebrating

Reflecting on her success, Amy shared:

"I would never trade your guidance and everything you've done for me over these past several months. It gave me a focused plan, exactly what I needed. I placed in every race this year. It worked. I'm grateful."

Amy's journey is a testament to the power of mindset. She didn't just finish her first 70.3—she embraced the process, stayed consistent, and achieved something she once thought impossible. Her story proves that it's never too late to start, and with the right support, anything is possible.

Solutions: Building Mental Resilience

1. **Visualization**: Mental imagery is a powerful tool. Athletes like Gaye use visualization to rehearse race-day scenarios. Picture yourself swimming confidently, cycling with strength, and running across the finish line. This mental preparation builds confidence and reduces anxiety.

2. **Positive Affirmations**: Reframe your inner dialogue. Replace thoughts like, "I'm too slow," with affirmations such as, "I'm improving every day." These small mental shifts have a compounding effect, reinforcing belief in your abilities.

3. **Celebrate Small Wins**: Big goals can feel overwhelming. Break them into smaller steps and celebrate each milestone. Whether it's swimming an extra lap or completing a challenging workout, acknowledging progress builds momentum.

4. **Trust the Process**: Progress isn't always linear. There will be setbacks, but staying committed to your plan and focusing on what you can control ensures steady improvement.

Tim's Story: Crushing Goals and Breaking Barriers at 57

After finishing his Chattanooga 70.3, Tim from Arkansas reached out to Feisty Fox Coaching with a big goal: to conquer the North Carolina 70.3 in under 6 hours. But self-doubt loomed. *"I'm nervous about the ocean swim,"* he admitted. *"I don't have access to the ocean or any experience racing in it. My bike isn't as strong, and I'm nervous about cramping on the run."*

Despite his concerns, Tim committed to the process. "If sub-6 hours is what you want, we'll get you there. We have 5 months" I told him. "Follow the plan, and you'll build the confidence you need."

Fast forward to race day: Tim didn't just meet his sub-6-hour goal—he crushed it, finishing in 5:39:19 at age 57, with personal records in all three sports. He even beat his PR from five years earlier. This transformation wasn't just physical; it was mental.

Overcoming Doubt and Learning to Believe

Tim's journey was about more than race times. He started with hesitations many athletes can relate to—fear of the unknown, doubts about his abilities, and questions about whether his age or lack of ocean swimming experience would hold him back. Through focused training, he built confidence step by step, learning to trust the process.

"I realized that every workout adds up over time," Tim reflects. *"It wasn't about doing everything perfectly—it was about showing up consistently, trusting my coach, and being open to feedback."*

The Turning Point: Trusting the Process

At Chattanooga, Tim struggled with cramps on the bike and run, realizing he needed to change his approach. By following the structured Feisty Fox Coaching plan, he learned to:

- **Dial in his pacing and cadence** to conserve energy for strong finishes.

- **Fine-tune his nutrition strategy,** eliminating cramps and guesswork.

- **Embrace direct feedback** that pushed him to improve, even when it was tough to hear.

"At first, the direct feedback 'pissed me off,'" Tim admits. "But I realized I needed that push. I don't want sugarcoating—I WANT RESULTS. That directness drove me to prove I could do it."

Breaking Mental Barriers

Tim's biggest breakthroughs weren't physical—they were mental. He learned to overcome self-doubt, quiet his inner critic, and focus on the present. *"The last three miles were mind over body,"* Tim recalls. *"I kept saying to myself, 'Stay within yourself and keep running.'"*

This mindset shift transformed how Tim approached not just racing, but training and life. *"I've learned to give myself grace when things don't go perfectly and to celebrate the small wins along the way,"* he says.

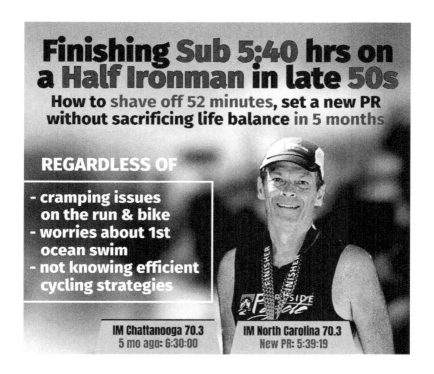

The Payoff: A New Perspective

Just four weeks after his 70.3 success, Tim smashed another personal record with a 1:43:13 finish at a half marathon with 1,200 feet of elevation gain, earning 2nd in his age group (55-59).

Now, he's setting even bigger goals—eyeing top-10 age group finishes and breaking the 5:30 barrier for 70.3 races.

Reflecting on his journey, Tim shares his top lessons:

1. **Consistency is Key:** *"You don't have to be perfect—just keep showing up. Every workout matters."*

2. **Trust Your Coach:** *"Feedback is what drives improvement,*

even when it's hard to hear."

3. **Celebrate the Journey:** *"It's not just about race day. The friendships, health, and joy training brings are worth it."*

Tim's story is proof that age, past setbacks, or self-doubt don't define your potential. With the right mindset, guidance, and commitment, you can achieve more than you ever thought possible. In just five months, Tim shattered his 70.3 personal record by almost an hour, applying his top lessons and following the Smart Training Method and 360 Strategic Training.

Where will you be five months from now?

Becoming World-Class with the Feisty Fox Mindset

Our vision is clear: To help triathletes become world-class in both their performance and their lives. A world-class athlete is someone who:

- **Balances** their passion for triathlon with their relationships, career, and health.

- **Adapts** to challenges with resilience and resourcefulness.

- **Trains** with purpose and prioritizes injury prevention and longevity.

- **Inspires** others by living their values and chasing their dreams.

Takeaways: How to Train Your Mind for Success

Just like your body, your mind needs regular training to grow stronger. Here's how to cultivate an unstoppable mindset:

- **Start Your Day with Intention**: Begin each morning with a positive affirmation or a quick visualization of your goals.

- **Focus on the Process**: Instead of fixating on the finish line, enjoy the journey of becoming stronger, fitter, and more confident.

- **Control the Controllable**: Accept what's out of your hands and channel your energy into what you can influence.

- **Celebrate Progress**: No win is too small. Every step forward is a step closer to your goals.

By embracing the Feisty Fox mindset, you're not just preparing for your next race—you're building a foundation for success in every area of your life.

Inspiration: A Call to Action

A Feisty Fox believes in themselves, even on the tough days. They know that **growth** lies on the other side of discomfort and that setbacks are just stepping stones to greatness.

So, the next time doubts creep in, remind yourself: "I am capable. I am resilient. I am becoming world-class."

Because when you commit to the journey, there's nothing you can't achieve. **You're not just a triathlete—you're a Feisty Fox.**

Chapter 7 Summary: *The Mindset of an Unstoppable Athlete*

Key Insight: The biggest challenges in triathlon aren't physical—they're mental. Success starts with adopting a resilient, growth-oriented mindset that turns doubts into fuel for progress.

Core Principles:

- **Consistency over Perfection:** Show up regularly; progress is built over time.

- **Intentional Training:** Every session has a purpose—focus on quality, not quantity.

- **Adaptability:** Life happens; adjust your training rather than abandoning it.

- **Growth-Oriented Thinking:** Treat setbacks as opportunities to learn and grow.

- **Positivity and Patience:** Celebrate small wins and stay focused on long-term progress.

Inspiration from Real Stories: Athletes like Gaye, Seiko, Amy and Tim transformed their mindset and achieved extraordinary results by focusing on resilience, recovery, and trusting the process. They proved that age, experience, or circumstances don't define your potential—your mindset does.

Actionable Steps for Cultivating an Unstoppable Mindset

- **Start Your Day with Intention:**

  - Use affirmations like, "I am resilient," or visualize yourself succeeding in a challenging workout or race.

- **Develop Body Awareness:**

  - Listen to your body. Differentiate between normal fatigue and pain. Adjust your training accordingly to prevent injury.

- **Embrace Visualization:**

  - Picture yourself conquering race-day challenges. Visualize transitions, strong strokes, or steady climbs to build confidence and reduce anxiety.

- **Reframe Negative Thoughts:**

  - Replace self-doubt with empowering affirmations. Shift "I'm too slow" to "I'm getting stronger every day."

- **Set Micro-Goals:**

  - Break big goals into smaller, manageable steps. Celebrate every milestone, whether it's completing an extra swim lap or shaving seconds off your pace.

- **Prioritize Recovery:**

  - Schedule rest days, focus on quality sleep, and incorporate active recovery to stay refreshed and injury-free.

- **Trust the Process:**

  - Acknowledge that progress isn't always linear. Stay consistent and focus on long-term growth, even when setbacks arise.

- **Build a Support Network:**

  - Surround yourself with like-minded athletes, coaches, or groups. Share your wins and challenges to stay motivated.

Reflection Questions to Deepen Your Mindset

1. What self-doubts or limiting beliefs are holding you back, and how can you reframe them positively?

2. What small, specific goals can you set this week to build momentum?

3. How can you practice adaptability when life disrupts your training plan?

4. What does success look like for you beyond race results?

5. Who inspires you, and how can you incorporate their mindset into your journey?

6. What's one way you can celebrate your progress this week, no matter how small?

7. How can you use visualization or affirmations to boost your confidence before a challenging workout or race?

By focusing on these steps and questions, you'll not only strengthen your mindset but also build a foundation for success in triathlon—and life.

Remember: being unstoppable isn't about being perfect; it's about showing up, learning, and growing every day.

SPECIAL GIFT for You! Free Access to My Training Video

Thank you for reading *Unstoppable: The Smart Training Method*! While this book gives you the tools to transform your training, this **free training video** takes it a step further.

What's Inside:

- The **5 Pillars** to train smarter, avoid injuries, and race strong.

- Real-life success stories and practical tips you can apply right away.

- How to troubleshoot challenges like missed workouts, motivation slumps, or injuries.

How Is This Different from this Book?

This video is like a personal coaching session—I'll walk you through strategies, examples, and solutions that go beyond what's in the book.

How to Access:

Scan the QR code below or visit linktr.ee/feistyfox.

SCAN ME

This is your next step to unstoppable success. Let's crush those goals together!

P.S. Watching this will save you years of trial and error—think of it as your shortcut to success.

Chapter 8

Your Next Steps

Congratulations! You've taken the time to explore how to balance your passion for triathlon with the demands of life, the fear of injury, and the constraints of time. But reading about it is just the beginning. Now, it's **time to take action**.

This chapter is about **empowering** you to move forward with confidence, knowing that you can achieve your triathlon goals without sacrificing your health, relationships, or life balance. Whether you're aiming to finish your first 70.3 or smash your personal record, the right guidance can make all the difference.

Why Feisty Fox Coaching Works

At Feisty Fox Coaching, we understand the unique challenges faced by busy achievers like you. Our approach is designed to fit seamlessly into your life, making triathlon training an enriching part of your routine—not an overwhelming burden. Here's what makes our method stand out:

1. Holistic Coaching for Long-Term Success

Triathlon isn't just about crossing the finish line; it's about integrating every aspect of your life to ensure long-term success. Our **Smart Training Method** focuses on:

- **Training:** Structured, purpose-driven sessions tailored to your goals.

- **Nutrition:** Optimized plans that fuel your performance and recovery.

- **Body Maintenance:** Injury prevention strategies and recovery routines to keep you feeling strong.

- **Mental Fitness:** Techniques to build resilience and confidence.

- **Race Strategy:** Personalized plans to ensure race-day success.

By addressing all five pillars, we help you stay injury-free, maintain balance, and achieve sustainable results.

2. Expert-Led Coaching and Community Support

At Feisty Fox Coaching, your performance doesn't rely on just one coach. You have access to a dedicated **team of experts** working together to support every aspect of your triathlon journey. Our team includes:

- **Triathlon Coaches** for tailored training plans and race strategies.

- **Sports Performance Psychologists** to build mental resilience and confidence.

- **Swim, Run and Bike Technique Experts & Gait Analysts** to optimize your technique and efficiency.

- **Physical Therapists** to prevent injuries and address recovery needs.

- **Registered Dietitians** to create personalized nutrition plans.

- **Injury Prevention Strategists** to keep you strong and injury-free.

- **Strength Trainers** for endurance-specific strength-building.

- **Yoga Instructors** to enhance flexibility and balance.

- **Athlete Success Specialists** serve as your accountability partners and tech-support go-to, ensuring you stay on track with the tools and resources needed to succeed.

You're not just getting a coach—you're gaining the support of an all-star team dedicated to helping you thrive in every area of your training and racing.

3. Customized Plans for Busy Achievers

Your life is unique, and your training plan should be, too. Whether you're a parent juggling family commitments, a professional managing a demanding career, or both, we tailor your program to fit your schedule and goals. From 10-hour training weeks to flexible indoor and outdoor options, we work with your reality—not against it.

4. A Proven System with Real Results

Feisty Fox Coaching is built on values that ensure longevity and success:

- **Injury-Free:** Prioritizing techniques that reduce strain and promote recovery.

- **Optimal Health:** Supporting your overall well-being beyond just race day.

- **Life Balance:** Helping you thrive in all areas of life, not just triathlon.

- **Longevity in Training and Racing:** Ensuring sustainable success.

- **Results-Driven:** Focused on tangible, measurable progress.

5. Proven Success Stories

Athletes of all ages and experience levels have trusted Feisty Fox Coaching to guide them to success.

- **Gwen:** A full-time working mom of five children aged 5 to 13, completed her first full Ironman at Arizona by creatively managing her time—training early mornings and averaging 10-11 hours a week. She prioritized her family without missing holidays, birthdays, or special moments, proving that smart training method and commitment make anything possible.

- **Kelly and Sarrah**: Two moms in their 40s balanced family, work, and triathlon training, inspiring their children while excelling in their own races. Sarrah motivated her son to work harder in soccer, while Kelly's kids started participating in races themselves, turning triathlon into a family passion.

- **Bob**: In his 60s, Bob overcame persistent knee pain and achieved personal bests through structured, life-aligned training. At 63, he ran a 1:40:44 half marathon and completed a 70.3 Ironman in 5:20:34, proving age is no barrier to peak performance.

- **Gaye**: A physical therapist who went from barely swimming to completing an Ironman in just 9 months, all while working full-time and managing family commitments. Her journey included PRs in the Berlin and London marathons and overcoming an IT band injury, proving that with the Smart Training Method and determination, self-doubt can be conquered.

- **Amy**: New to triathlon at 55, Amy completed her first 70.3 at Ironman 70.3 Muncie, placed 9th in her age group, and qualified for the World Championship in Spain. Her success came from trusting the process, dialing in her nutrition, and sharing the experience with her family.

- **Zo:** A 58-year-old CrossFit trainer, yoga instructor, and water aerobics coach, Zo overcame 7 weeks of chronic heel pain through personalized injury-free training. By addressing her run technique, balancing stress and recovery, and prioritizing body maintenance, she podiumed & ran total 100 miles in a month pain-free.

- **Tim:** At 57, Tim shaved 52 minutes off his 70.3 time, smashed his sub-6-hour goal with 5h 39m while setting PRs in all three disciplines. His mental breakthroughs and dedication prove that age is just a number.

- **Erik**: A dad of four and business owner, Erik achieved his dream of qualifying for Ironman World Championship Kona on his 2nd Ironman by balancing training, work, and family. His focus on mental resilience, trusting his coach, and building a strong community were key to his success.

- **Reggie**: A business owner and father of three, Reggie trained 80% indoors and completed his first full Ironman at Arizona despite frequent travel and limited outdoor training. By involving his family in the journey, he turned the experience into a shared victory.

- **Scott**: A resilient athlete with a history of injuries, including plantar fasciitis, knee pain, and hip issues, Scott transformed his training approach to focus on root causes instead of symptoms. By strengthening stabilizer muscles, improving alignment, and balancing his workload, he achieved remarkable milestones: a 70.3 PR of 5:37:48, a Boston Marathon qualifier of 3:06:15, and his first full Ironman finish in 11:30:16—all in one year. Scott's journey proves that addressing imbalances and training smarter can unlock extraordinary achievements.

- **Seiko:** A busy woman in her late 40s with limited swim access, Seiko qualified for both the full Ironman and 70.3 World Championships. Her focus on recovery, visualization, and personalized nutrition helped her excel despite a demanding schedule.

- **Jeremy:** A busy father with no prior swimming or cycling experience, Jeremy went from struggling to complete a single pool lap to finishing his first full Ironman within seven months. Through structured training, smart nutrition, and unwavering consistency, he overcame cramping issues and a hectic schedule. Within a year, Jeremy also completed an 8.2-mile open-water swim and inspired his family with his remarkable transformation. His story proves that with effort and commitment, no challenge is too big

- **Justin:** A father of four and busy business owner, Justin finished his first Ironman in 12:51:14, setting PRs in both 70.3 and half marathon distances, all while managing past knee injuries and staying injury-free.

- **Leo:** A veteran who faced an extraordinary journey through multiple surgeries, PTSD, and chronic pain, Leo rebuilt his strength and confidence by training smarter, not harder. He completed two (2) Ironman races, proving that resilience and a smart plan can overcome even the toughest obstacles.

These stories are proof that with the right coaching, anything is possible—even for busy, high-achieving individuals like you.

6. Empowering a Supportive Community

When you join Feisty Fox Coaching, you become part of a vibrant, driven **community of athletes** who:

- Share insights and experiences to keep each other motivated.

- Celebrate wins, both big and small, to keep the momentum going.

- Create a camaraderie that turns individual achievements into shared victories.

7. A Clear Path to Your Goals

Every workout, recovery plan, and mental strategy is designed to get you one step closer to your goals. With structured guidance, expert support, and a focus on building confidence, we ensure you're always moving forward.

Your Call to Action

Now that you've seen what's possible, the next step is up to you. Imagine crossing the finish line of your race, stronger and more confident than ever before.

Picture yourself balancing your training, work, and family life seamlessly, all while staying injury-free. That vision is within reach, and we're here to help you make it a reality.

Here's what you can do next:

Take Your Journey Even Further. Scan the QR Code Below to:

1. **Unlock exclusive Unstoppable book resources** to:

   a. Level up your swim, bike, run, and time management skills by applying the Smart Training Method and 360 Strategic Training tools from this book.

   b. Be inspired by real-life stories from athletes who overcame challenges, found solutions, and crushed their biggest goals.

   c. Dive deeper with step-by-step guidance through our coaching programs, tailored to help you implement these strategies into your life.

2. **Schedule a 15-minute Game Plan Call** to discuss your personal goals, identify the first steps to get you closer to achieving them and receive actionable advice tailored just for you.

Your best self - the strongest, healthiest and most empowered version of yourself is waiting. Let's get started.

RESERVE A
15 MIN
GAMEPLAN

SCAN ME

GET MORE
RESOURCES
SCAN ME

Inspiration

Why settle for average when you can achieve greatness? No matter your background, past struggles, or current challenges, you have the power to rewrite your story and accomplish the impossible.

This book is filled with real-life stories of athletes who, like you, once doubted their potential. They took the first step, committed to the process, and achieved what they once thought was out of reach.

As I always say: ***"Dream big, take action. Anything is possible. With the right mindset, smart strategies, and unwavering determination, we can break barriers, defy limits, and achieve greatness beyond what we imagined. Why settle for average when you can be your best?"***

Let's make your dreams a reality. Together, we'll push boundaries, shatter limits, and achieve greatness—without sacrificing the joy of living your best life.

Ready to Begin?

Schedule Your Free Game Plan call Now.

Let's get started on your journey to **becoming** the best version of yourself.

Your next finish line is waiting.

SCAN ME

RESERVE A 15 MIN GAMEPLAN

About the author

As a 2x Guinness World Record holder in triathlon, a best-selling author, and a performance coach with over 20 years of experience, Shangrila has helped thousands of athletes achieve their biggest goals—from finishing their first sprint triathlon, marathons to qualifying for the Boston Marathon, Ironman Kona, ultra endurance and other prestigious races.

But it wasn't always this way. Shangrila started from a place many can relate to: no background in swimming, cycling, or running, and overwhelmed by the challenges of a busy life. While working full-time as an engineer in the medical device industry, she discovered triathlon as a path to healing from 26 years of childhood abuse, addiction, sexual assault, PTSD, and an eating disorder. Determined to succeed despite her limitations, she immersed herself in learning and developed a smarter approach to training—one that worked even for someone juggling demanding careers, personal struggles, and time constraints.

Her credentials are as comprehensive as her journey. She is certified in advanced swim technique, run gait analysis, cycling power training, TRX strength training, yoga instruction, and injury prevention methods. Shangrila has applied these skills not only to her own racing career—completing 48 Ironman races, Ironman Kona, Ultraman and cycling across America—but also to creating the Feisty Fox Smart Training Method, a proven system built on science, experience, and real-world testing.

Shangrila knows firsthand the struggles busy high achievers face: not enough time, fear of injury, and the challenge of maintaining life balance.

Her method isn't about training harder; it's about training smarter—maximizing every minute to deliver peak performance while staying injury-free. With her expertise, you'll gain more than a training plan; you'll gain the confidence to redefine what's possible.As featured in *The New York Times*, *Triathlete Magazine*, Outside Magazine, 220 Triathlon Magazine, Red Bull TV, Fox, CBS, and NBC news, Shangrila continues to inspire and equip athletes to transform their lives, one smart step at a time.

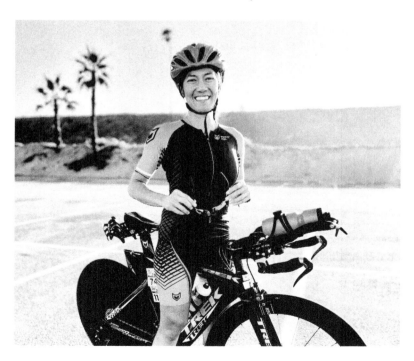

How to contact Shangrila Rendon

For more information about coaching, keynote and workshops, contact Feisty Fox Coaching

Online: www.feistyfoxcoaching.com

Phone: +1 405-679-2663

Email: support@feistyfoxcoaching.com

Feisty Fox Coaching

1110 N Virgil Ave Unit #91186 Los Angeles, CA 90029

Printed in Great Britain
by Amazon